the
naked
diet

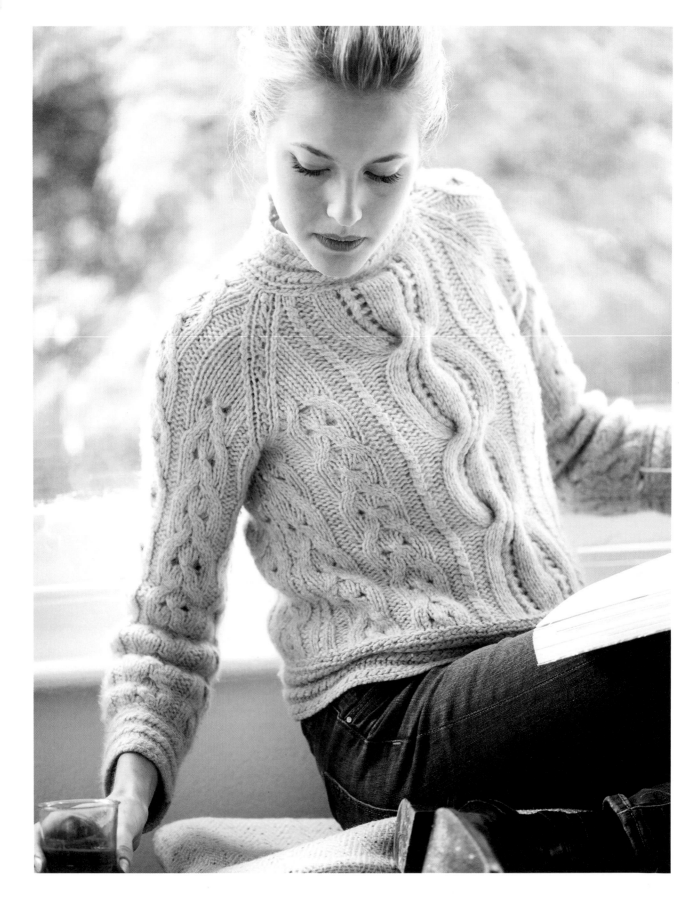

the naked diet

tess ward

photography by columbus leth

QUADRILLE

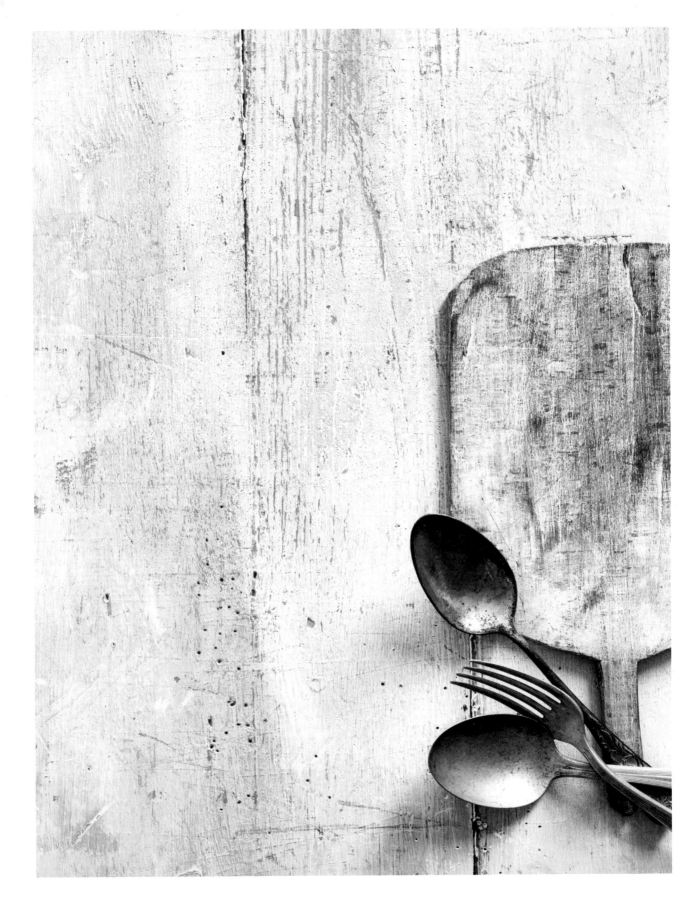

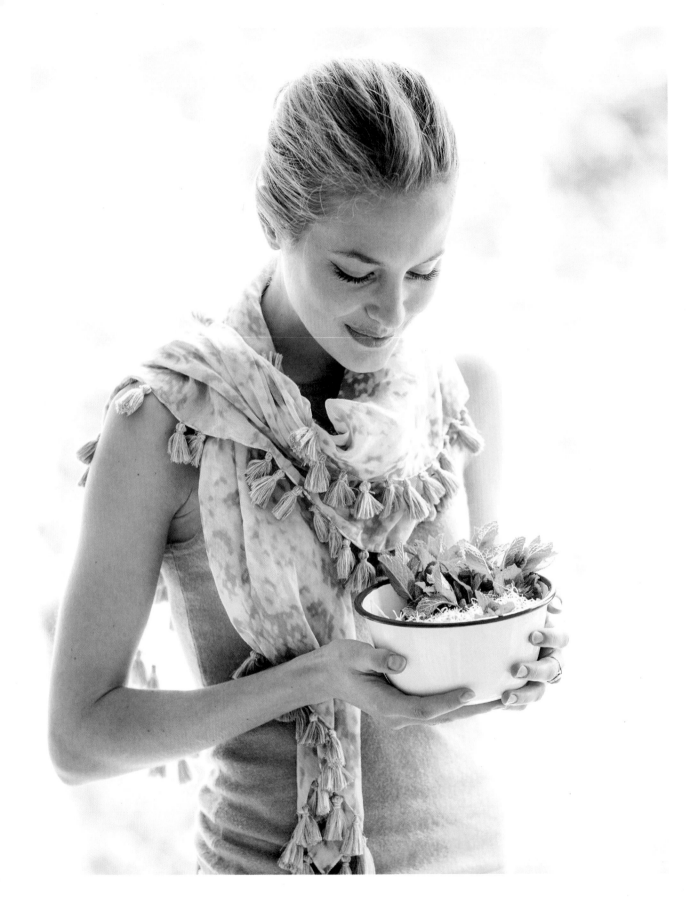

introduction

the idea

Over the years the word 'diet' as we understand it has changed. **the naked diet's** interpretation is based on the Latin origins of the word 'diata', meaning 'way of life'. To me a diet is exactly that. Not a quick fix, but a sustained way of eating that naturally supports our overall health and happiness.

Few people I know would claim that they follow their ideal diet, although this seems to be what everyone aspires to. Many of us still subscribe to the idea of 'diet' in the short term, and its promise to change, help or improve us. Lose the tummy, have slimmer thighs, a tighter bum, because it will make us happier, right? Why else diet other than to improve our quality of life in some way. So many of these unrealistic regimes claim to do this and they may well succeed in the short term. But anything beyond the initial 'starve yourself for a few weeks and lose weight', goes uncovered. In fact, any form of longevity is pretty much ignored, meaning the dieter ultimately ends up at the bottom of the heap, feeling worse than they did before they started. Too many diets are based too heavily in theory and not in practice. What works for one person is completely different for another. Nutrition and diet is an area full of contradictory information and evidence, there simply isn't a 'perfect diet', or 'one diet that fits all'; instead, it's about finding the best balance in one's own body.

The most important thing is to have a balanced understanding of what our own body truly needs. **the naked diet** moves away from processed and refined foods, unrealistic diets and fad regimes, instead it is about eating food in its most naked form.

my experience

A year ago, a restricted diet was something I was all too familiar with. Not for weight, but for health reasons. Aged 18, I spent a month travelling in India. On the way I picked up a parasite, that I was to live with for the next five years. Over this period there were repeat visits to doctors and specialists. I was diagnosed with post-infectious IBS, given more antibiotics than a dairy cow, and put on a restrictive diet. It wasn't until I met Humphrey Bacchus, a clinical nutritionist and medicine practitioner, who finally diagnosed my problem.

The recipes in this book are a compilation of the foods I have uncovered and created on my journey back to full health. The recipes have been designed to support and fuel your body, encourage optimal health, through simple, delicious and stripped back recipes.

this book

This book is all about eating food in its purest form. **the naked diet** celebrates creativity in cooking and all the recipes are efficient, practical and packed full of taste. They have been inspired by all the wonderful chefs I have worked with and the countries, cuisines and restaurants I have been to. I hope you find my naked dishes as pleasurable to make, eat and use as I have found discovering and creating them.

Cook naked, eat happy and you'll never have to do the dreaded 'diet' again.

naked broths + stocks

Broth is typically made with bones, and can contain a small amount of meat adhering to the bones. As with stock, bones are typically roasted first to improve the flavour of the broth, which is simmered for a long period of time (often in excess of 24 hours) whereas stock is simmered for 3–4 hours. Broth's long cooking time helps to extract as many minerals and nutrients as possible from the bones. At the end of cooking, the minerals have leached from the bones into the broth and the bones crumble when pressed between your thumb and forefinger.

broth's goodness

Broths are extraordinarily rich in nutrients – particularly minerals and amino acids, especially arginine, glycine and proline. Glycine supports the body's detoxification process and is used in the synthesis of haemoglobin, bile salts and other naturally occurring chemicals within the body, as well as supporting digestion and the secretion of gastric acids. Proline, especially when paired with vitamin C, supports good skin health.

Bone broths are also rich in gelatin, which improves collagen status, that supports skin health and also aids digestive health.

stock's goodness

Stocks are also typically made with bones, they contain a small amount of meat and are typically simmered for less time than a broth, 3–4 hours. Stock is rich in both minerals and gelatin.

Chicken stock inhibits neutrophil migration; it helps mitigate the side effects of colds, flu and upper respiratory infections.

basic roast chicken stock/broth

1 leftover roast chicken carcass
vegetable scraps (celery leaves, onion trimmings, leeks, fennel, carrot peelings, garlic etc)
2 bay leaves
few thyme sprigs
handful of parsley stalks

for asian chicken stock/broth:
5cm piece of fresh ginger
1 star anise
3–4 fresh cayenne (or other) chilli peppers
unpeeled cloves of 1 whole garlic bulb, bashed
10cm lemongrass stalk (optional)

1 Put the chicken carcass, vegetable scraps and herbs into a stockpot or for asian stock/broth omit the vegetables and herbs and add the asian ingredients.

2 Pour in enough cold water to cover the carcass by about 5cm, about 1 litre. Cover, bring to the boil, then reduce the heat to low and simmer for 3 hours (for stock) or for 24 hours or longer (for broth), adding water now and then if making broth until the bones become flexible and rubbery, and skimming off any scum that rises to the top, from time to time.

3 Strain through a fine mesh sieve and pour into jars. The broth should gel, but it is not necessary. Store in the fridge for 2–3 days, or decant into freezer containers and freeze for up to 1 month.

makes about 800ml

beef stock/broth

Roasting the bones ensures a good flavour in the resulting beef stock. If making soup, it's wise to serve this stock very hot as it may gel once it cools.

2.8–3kg grass-fed beef bones
vegetable scraps
2–3 bay leaves
few thyme sprigs
couple of rosemary sprigs

1 Preheat the oven to 200°C/ Gas Mark 6. Rinse the bones, dry and spread in a roasting tin (they should fit in a single layer).

2 Roast for about 1 hour, then remove from the oven and drain off any fat. Add the bones to a stockpot along with vegetable scraps. Add cold water to cover, about 1 litre, cover, bring to the boil and add the herbs. Turn down the heat and simmer, covered, for at least 3 hours (for stock) and up to 24 hours (for broth), skimming off any foam.

3 Strain through a mesh sieve and pour into jars. The stock should set like gelatin and the fat should rise to the top. Remove the fat and reserve for cooking. To serve as soup, scoop out the gelled stock and reheat.

4 Store in the fridge for 2–3 days, or decant into freezer containers and freeze for up to 1 month.

makes about 800ml

fish stock

The best fish bones for stock are from fine fish – ask your fishmonger to remove the gills behind the cheek flaps to prevent any bitterness. Don't use the bones of oily fish. This is not as extravagant as it sounds, as fishmongers will often hand over the bones for free.

500g fish bones
1 carrot, 1 celery stick,
and 1 onion, all chopped into
pea-sized pieces
parsley stalks and fennel bulb
trimmings (optional)
1 bay leaf

1 Put all the ingredients into a stockpot and add cold water to cover by an inch. Cover, bring to the boil and spoon off any white or grey froth that settles on the surface. Reduce the heat and simmer, covered, for 20–25 minutes.

2 Strain through a fine mesh sieve into a bowl, leave to cool.

3 Store in the fridge for 2–3 days, or decant into freezer containers and freeze for up to 1 month.

makes 1.5–2 litres

miso soup

Miso soup is a traditional Japanese broth made from fermented soya beans. It is high in manganese, copper and zinc and is a good source of protein and dietary fibre. As a fermented food, it is also beneficial to digestive health. The micro-organisms used in fermentation of soy miso can actively help metabolise proteins, carbohydrates and fats, transforming them into smaller more easily digested molecules.

1 litre water
1 sachet bonito fish stock,
or dashi
2–3 tablespoons miso paste
2 spring onions, finely chopped

optional extras:
1 tablespoon shredded nori or
wakame seaweed
½ block of firm silken tofu, cut
into 2.5cm cubes

1 Bring the water to a simmer in a pan and add the seaweed (if using). Simmer for 5 minutes, then reduce the heat to very low and add the remaining ingredients. Stir until the miso is well dissolved, then remove from the heat. Don't let the miso boil, as it kills the beneficial nutrients and alters the soup's flavour. Serve hot.

serves 4

naked infused oils

The quality of the oil you select depends on what you want to use it for. For instance, if you are making a chilli oil to use as a condiment, then use a high-quality extra virgin. But if you are just intending to cook with it, then a more basic olive oil is more suitable.

It is important to use dried rather than fresh ingredients, such as herbs and chillies, to infuse your oil. Fresh spices and herbs release moisture that can cause bacteria to form in the oil (the only exception being garlic). If you are going to include ingredients with any potential moisture into your infusions, make sure you dry them out completely before using. It is also important to sterilise the jars before use.

To make the infused oils last longer, you can heat it with the infusing ingredients, which kills any bacteria. To do this, combine the oil and herbs in a small saucepan and place over a low heat for about 5 minutes, until the oil gets hot (but don't let it boil). Remove from the heat, cover, and leave to cool to room temperature. Transfer the herbs to a sterilised bottle, then add the oil. Seal and keep for 2–3 months.

However, don't heat extra virgin oil as it damages the quality and the health benefits of the oil. Although this means this kind of infused oil won't last as long (around 2–3 weeks), you can just reduce the quantities of it that you make.

For these infused oils (pictured opposite), use 500ml extra virgin or olive oil.

chilli oil
(pictured top left on opposite page)

10–20 small dried red chillies

garlic oil
(pictured bottom left on opposite page)

**6 garlic cloves, peeled
and halved**

rosemary + bay oil
(pictured top right on opposite page)

**2 large rosemary sprigs
4 bay leaves**

lemon + pink peppercorn oil
(pictured bottom right on opposite page)

**pared strips of zest of 2 lemons
2 tablespoons pink
peppercorns**

1 Leave the pared zest to dry in a warm place for 1 week before using. Or use the oil heating method.

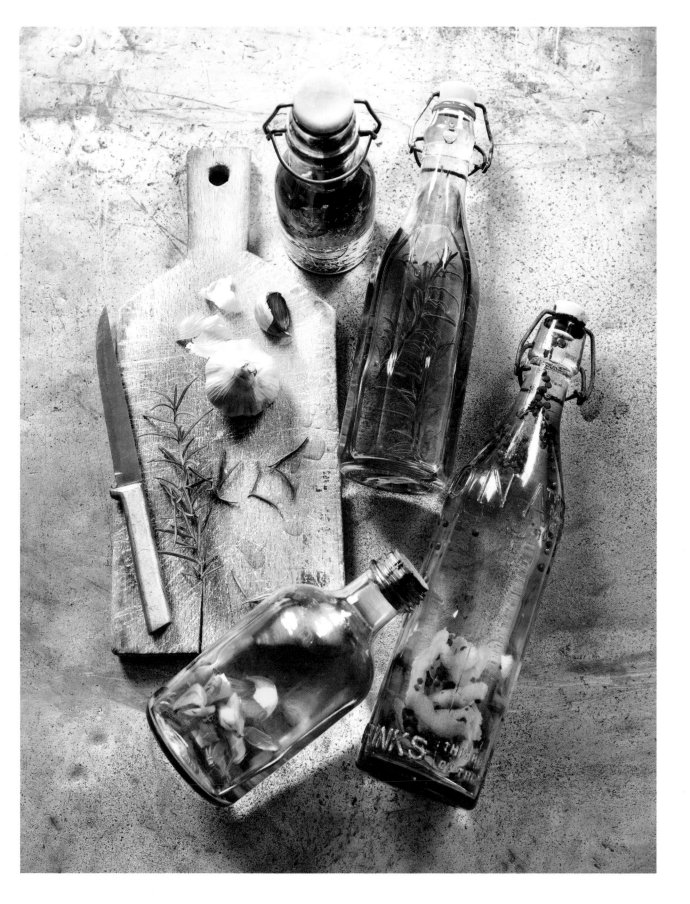

naked dips

easy goat's milk ricotta

(pictured top left on opposite page)

I have a bit of a bee in my bonnet about shop-bought ricotta. Firstly, it is almost always rubbery, and secondly there is never an organic option. Since it is so easy to make, I do it myself. I would recommend using a thermometer, but you can do it by eye – just watch the milk like a hawk!

500ml full cream goat's (or buffalo) milk, ideally organic
¼ teaspoon fine sea salt
2 tablespoons lemon juice

1 Line a colander with 4 layers of muslin or 2 layers of food-safe kitchen paper, and set the colander over a large bowl.

2 Put the milk, salt and lemon juice in a saucepan and bring to the boil over a 70°C heat, stirring constantly. At this point the milk should begin to split, separating into solid white curds and translucent liquid whey. If only half the milk is curdling, add a few more drops of lemon juice.

3 Using a slotted spoon, transfer the separated curds to the lined colander, cover it with cling film and leave to drain for a few minutes if you like it quite soft, or for longer if you want it firmer.

4 Discard the liquid whey and store the ricotta in a sealed container in the fridge for up to 5 days.

makes 200ml

wasabi crème fraîche

(pictured bottom right on opposite page)

A dollop of wasabi is all that is needed to make this simple condiment exciting, as it adds a mustardy kick to any dish.

6 heaped tablespoons crème fraîche
2 teaspoons wasabi paste

1 Mix the crème fraîche with the wasabi paste in a small bowl or jar. Cover and store in the fridge for a week or so.

makes 80–100ml

coconut salsa

(pictured top right on opposite page + page 27)

This spicy salsa makes an ideal accompaniment to warming soups. For a dairy-free version, swap the Greek yoghurt for coconut yoghurt (see page 83).

150g desiccated coconut
400g thick, Greek-style yoghurt
10g coriander leaves, chopped
1 long green chilli, deseeded and finely chopped
1 teaspoon lime juice
½ teaspoon sea salt

1 Place the desiccated coconut in a bowl with 3–4 tablespoons hot water and leave to soften for 5 minutes. When the water has absorbed, mix the rest of the ingredients into the bowl.

makes 400–500ml

cucumber, radish + goat's cheese raita

(pictured bottom left on opposite page)

The goat's cheese adds a creamy richness to the raita, making it perfect as a condiment and side dip, but also as a filling for wraps, like the gluten-free crêpes (see page 80). A little tip: slice open the garlic and remove the germ (the little green piece inside the garlic); this will stop the garlic repeating on you when you eat it raw.

1 large cucumber, halved lengthways and deseeded
400g thick, Greek-style yoghurt
150g fresh goat's cheese
1 large garlic clove, finely chopped
juice of ½ lemon
200g fresh, firm radishes, very finely sliced
3 tablespoons chopped mint leaves
fine sea salt and freshly ground black pepper

1 Slice each deseeded cucumber and half very finely.

2 Place the yoghurt in a bowl and, using the back of a fork, mash in the goat's cheese. Gently fold in the cucumber, garlic, lemon juice, half the radishes and the mint and season with a generous pinch of salt and pepper. Top with the remaining radishes and serve.

makes 400–500ml

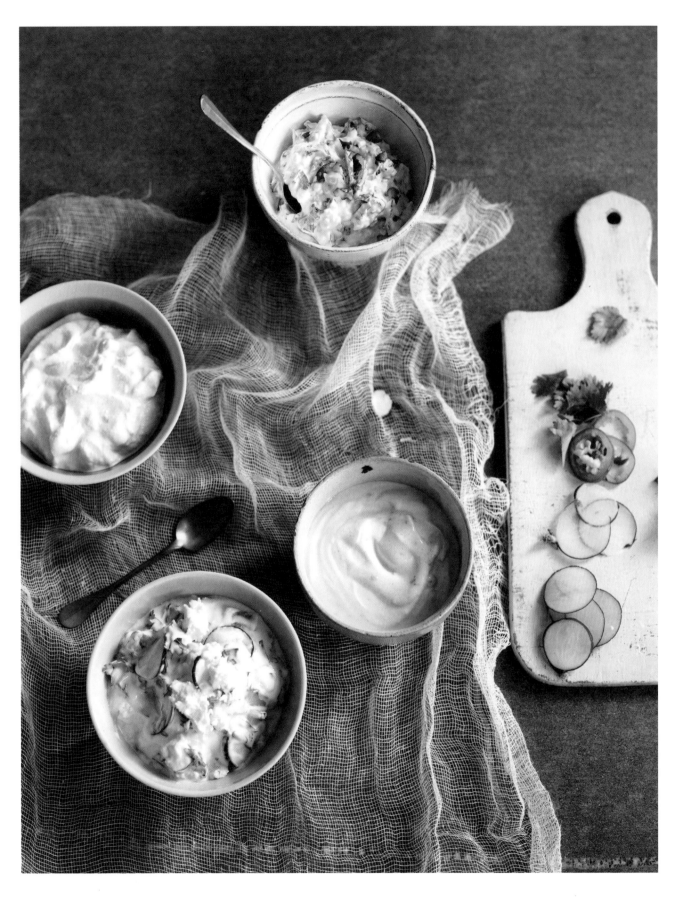

naked yoghurts

basil yoghurt dressing

Mix all the ingredients together in a small bowl, adding salt and pepper to taste.

1½ tablespoons plain
    probiotic yoghurt
4 tablespoons basil leaves,
    finely chopped
4 tablespoons extra virgin
    olive oil
2 tablespoons apple cider
    vinegar
2 teaspoons maple syrup
2 garlic cloves, mashed to
    a pulp
sea salt and freshly ground
    black pepper

makes 250ml

cumin yoghurt dressing

Whisk all the ingredients together in a small bowl, adding salt and pepper to taste.

3 tablespoons plain probiotic
    yoghurt
1 garlic clove, finely chopped
1 tablespoon cider vinegar
½ teaspoon honey
2 tablespoons olive oil
1 teaspoon cumin seeds,
    toasted and crushed
pinch of ground coriander
sea salt and freshly ground
    black pepper

makes 250ml

coriander yoghurt dressing

Mix all the ingredients together in a small bowl, adding salt and pepper to taste.

5 tablespoons thick,
    Greek-style yoghurt
2 tablespoons coriander
    leaves, chopped
½ teaspoon cumin seeds,
    toasted and crushed
1 teaspoon maple syrup
1 teaspoon lemon juice
1 garlic clove, finely chopped
1 teaspoon extra virgin olive oil
sea salt and freshly ground
    black pepper

makes 250ml

sauces

chunky peanut dipping sauce

3 tablespoons unsalted,
   chunky peanut butter
2 teaspoons toasted sesame oil
2 tablespoons soy sauce
2 teaspoons apple cider
   vinegar
1 tablespoon runny honey
juice of 1 orange

1 Put all the ingredients into a jar
and shake well.

2 Spoon into a bowl before
serving.

serves 2

thai dipping sauce

1 tablespoon toasted
   sesame oil
2 tablespoons lime juice
   (1–2 limes)
2 tablespoons fish sauce
1 red chilli, finely chopped
1½–2 tablespoons honey

1 Whisk the ingredients together
in a glass.

2 Spoon into a bowl before
serving.

serves 2–4

red cacao sauce

1 tablespoon coconut oil
½ teaspoon ground cumin
½ teaspoon spicy smoked
   paprika
1 onion, finely chopped
2 garlic cloves, finely
   chopped
220g tin tomatoes
8 coriander stalks, chopped
1 pitted date
1 tablespoon raw cacao
   powder
1 tablespoon smooth
   cashew nut butter
1 tablespoon lime juice
sea salt and freshly ground
   black pepper

1 To make the sauce, melt the
coconut oil in a frying pan, add
the cumin and paprika and cook,
stirring frequently. This should
take a couple of minutes. Add the
onion and a couple pinches of salt
and cook until softened. Add the
garlic and cook for another couple
of minutes.

2 Add the tomatoes and cook
for 5 minutes, then season and
transfer to a blender. Add the
coriander stalks, date, cacao
powder, cashew nut butter, lime
juice and 2 tablespoons of the
reserved poaching liquid. Blend
on high, adding more poaching
liquid to achieve the desired
consistency.

serves 2

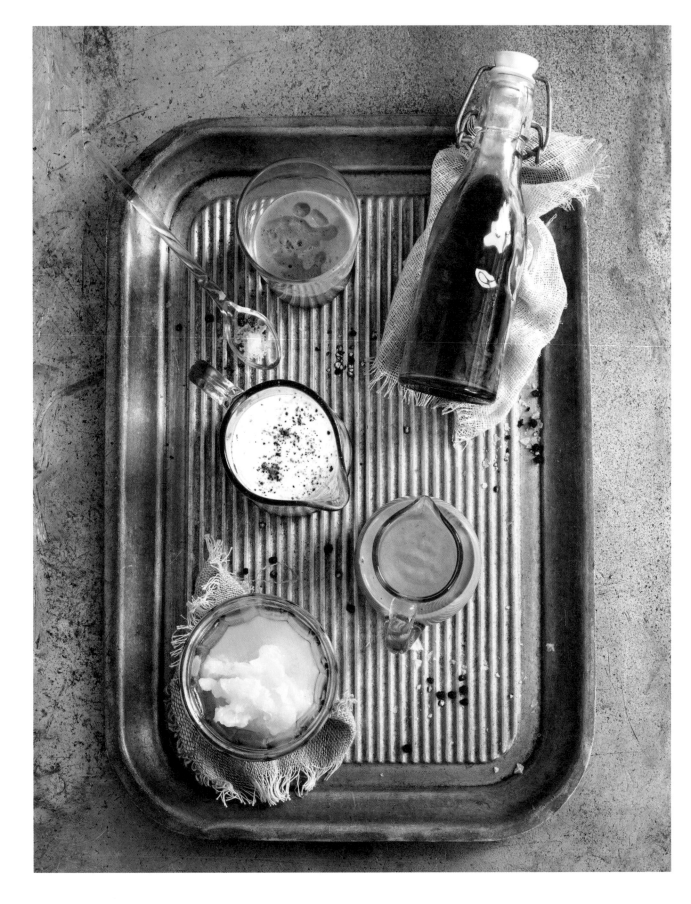

naked dressings

Possibly more vital than the dish itself is the dressing. Whether you are pouring, dipping, drizzling or using them as a condiment, it is great to have a selection in your repertoire. I often keep a couple of jars of my different naked dressings in the fridge for speedy use. For all dressings (barring the ghee) put the ingredients into a small jar, put a lid on and shake well to mix, then season to taste.

tamari dressing

(pictured bottom right on opposite page)

3 tablespoons tamari
2 tablespoons apple cider
  vinegar
finely grated zest and juice of
  1 lime
1 tablespoon honey
½ garlic clove, finely chopped
pinch of finely grated fresh
  ginger
1 tablespoon toasted sesame oil

makes 80–100ml

tahini dressing

(pictured middle left on opposite page)

2 tablespoons tahini
2 tablespoons tamari
2 tablespoons apple cider
  vinegar
finely grated zest and juice
  of 1 orange
½ garlic clove, finely chopped
1 teaspoon finely grated
  fresh ginger
1 tablespoon toasted
  sesame oil

makes 80–100ml

anchovy vinaigrette

(pictured top left on opposite page)

5 anchovies in olive oil,
  mashed with the side
  of a knife
1 teaspoon finely grated
  orange zest
2 teaspoons Dijon mustard
2 teaspoons apple cider
  vinegar
½ teaspoon honey
4 tablespoons extra virgin
  olive oil
sea salt and freshly ground
  black pepper

makes 80–100ml

honey balsamic dressing

(pictured top right on opposite page)

4 tablespoons extra virgin
  olive oil
2 tablespoons balsamic vinegar
1 teaspoon Dijon mustard
1 teaspoon honey (optional)
sea salt and freshly ground
  black pepper

makes 80–100ml

naked dressing

1 teaspoon grainy mustard
4 tablespoons orange juice
4 tablespoons extra virgin
  olive oil
sea salt and freshly ground
  black pepper

makes 80–100ml

homemade ghee

(pictured bottom left on opposite page)

500g unsalted, organic
  grass-fed butter

1 Sterilise a large jam jar by sitting it in a saucepan filled with enough water to submerge it. Bring the water to the boil, then drain and leave the jar to dry completely before using.

2 Heat the butter in a medium saucepan over a low heat. Once completely melted, simmer for 15–25 minutes, skimming off any froth that rises to the surface, until the milk solids begin to separate from the oil and sink to the bottom of the pan.

3 Remove from the heat and leave to cool for 15 minutes, then pour through a fine strainer or muslin-lined sieve into the sterilised jar, to remove the milk solids (discard these). Store in the fridge for up to 6 months.

makes 1 large jar

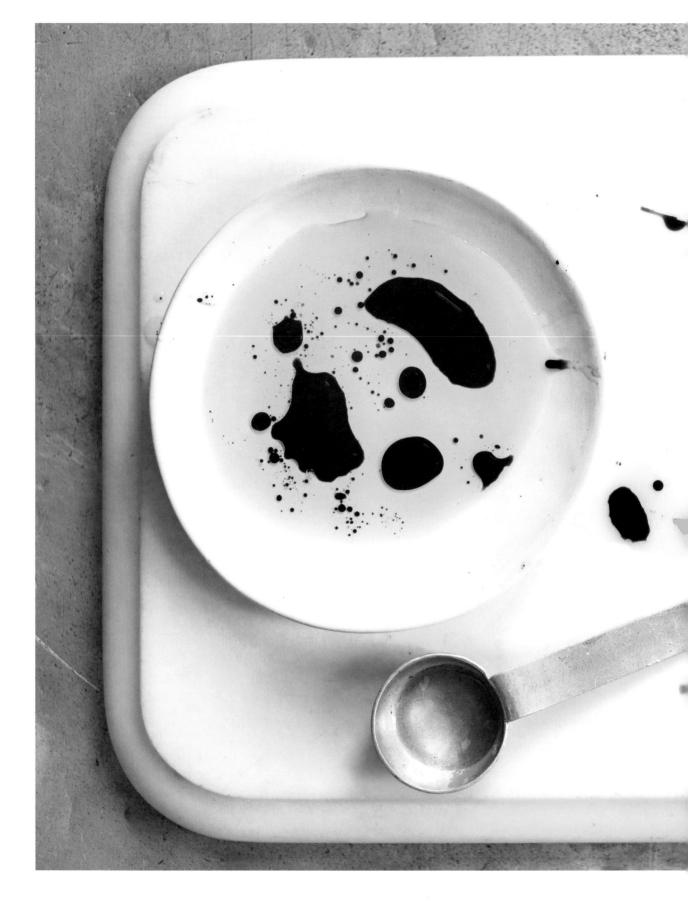

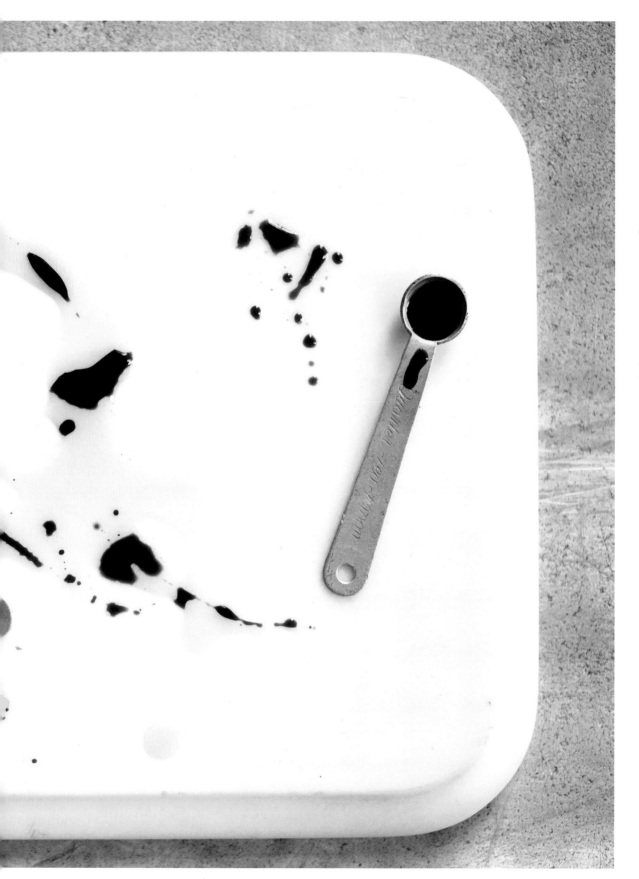

pure raw stripped bare nude clean detox

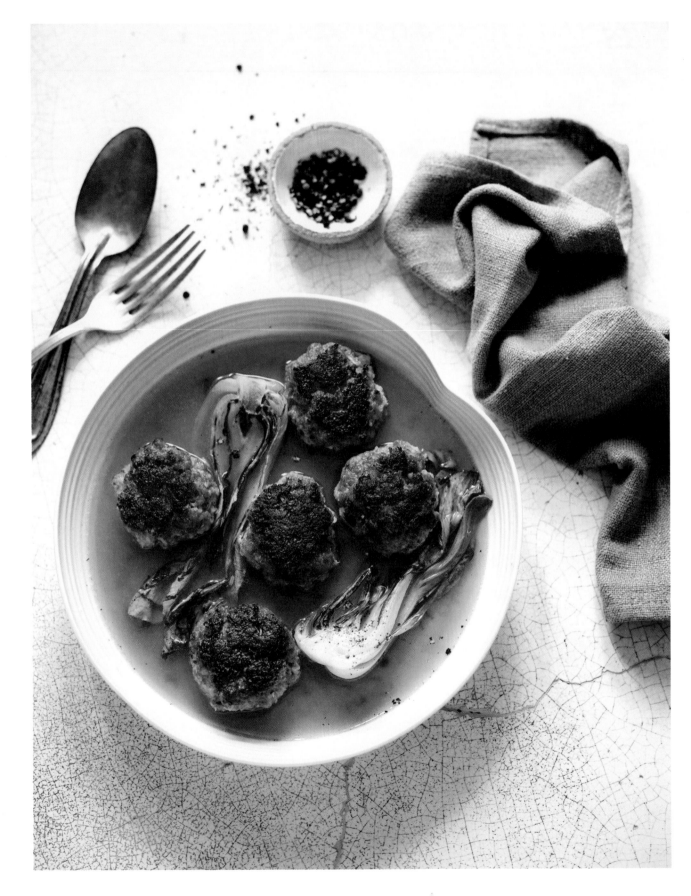

molasses + ginger porkballs with pak choi

Baked meatballs are a bit of a revelation; they acheive a pleasing oven-roasted crispness on top, but they are soft and mouthwateringly tender underneath.

500g pork mince
100g fresh rye or spelt
  breadcrumbs
3 garlic cloves,
  finely chopped
1 tablespoon grated
  fresh ginger
finely grated zest of
  1 lemon
1 heaped teaspoon spicy
  smoked paprika
2 tablespoons finely
  chopped coriander stalks
1 tablespoon blackstrap
  molasses
1 tablespoon honey
1 heaped teaspoon sea salt
freshly ground black
  pepper
1 tablespoon coconut oil,
  plus extra for the pak choi
600–800ml chicken
  stock (see page 8)
4 pak choi, halved

serves 2–3

1 Preheat the oven to 200°C/Gas Mark 6.

2 Put the pork mince, breadcrumbs, garlic, ginger, lemon zest and paprika in a mixing bowl. Add the coriander stalks, molasses, honey, salt and a little pepper. Using your hands, mix together well and then form the mixture into 12–14 balls or patties.

3 Heat the oil in a large frying pan, then fry the patties until brown on both sides. Place in a shallow ovenproof dish and add enough stock to come three quarters of the way up the patties. Cook in the oven for 15 minutes.

4 Meanwhile, heat a little oil in the pan used to cook the patties. Add the pak choi sliced side down and fry for a couple of minutes, adding a tablespoon of water halfway through to prevent burning till they are golden and soft.

5 Ladle the porkballs and cooking stock into shallow bowls, add the pak choi and a grinding of pepper, and serve.

bacon, cabbage + pearl barley broth

This simple, quick recipe is filling and cheap, as well as an ideal way to use up leftovers. The key is to use high-quality, strong-flavoured stock, preferably homemade. If you are short of time, you can use the cheaty pre-cooked packets of pearl barley, or mixed grains that are available in most supermarkets, just wash them first.

200g pearl barley
200g smoked bacon
    lardons
1 onion, finely chopped
1 large celery stalk, sliced
    into rounds (save the
    leaves for garnish)
4 garlic cloves, chopped
750ml chicken stock
    (see page 8)
½ small red cabbage, cut
    into shreds
small handful of flat-leaf
    parsley leaves
lemon juice, to taste
25g lightly toasted flaked
    almonds, to garnish
    (optional)
sea salt and freshly ground
    black pepper

serves 4

1 Put the pearl barley in a large saucepan, cover with cold water, add a big pinch of salt and bring to the boil. Reduce the heat to low, cover and simmer until the barley is cooked, 30–40 minutes, or according to the packet instructions. Drain well and return to the pan.

2 Meanwhile, cook the lardons in a frying pan over a high heat for 5 minutes, then add the onion and celery. Reduce the heat and gently sweat until soft. Add the garlic and cook for a couple of minutes, then tip the contents of the frying pan into the pan with the drained pearl barley.

3 Add the stock and bring to the boil, then reduce the heat and add the cabbage. Simmer for a further 10 minutes, or until the cabbage has softened but still retains texture and crunch. Season to taste.

4 Mix through the parsley and finish with a good squeeze of lemon. Ladle into bowls and enjoy hot, with a few celery leaves and a sprinkle of flaked almonds on top, if desired.

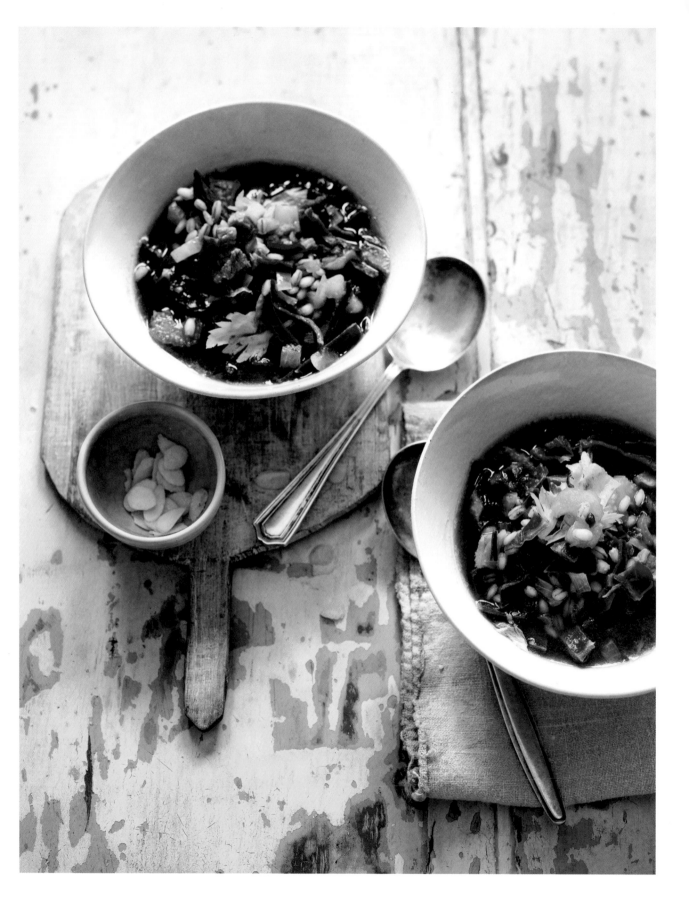

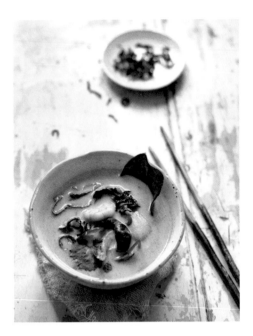

hot + spicy seafood soup with crispy shallots

This dish is a quicker, Thai fish-inspired version of my mother's magic, spicy coconut soup. It's warming, restorative and healing, with an added kick of chilli, zesty lime, lemongrass and ginger to clear the pipes and heat the belly.

2 tablespoons coconut oil

3 shallots, finely sliced

500ml chicken or fish stock

300ml coconut milk

1 heaped tablespoon tom
  yum paste

2.5cm piece of fresh ginger,
  grated

2 large fresh, or 4 dried,
  lime leaves

2 lemongrass stalks,
  bashed

75g shiitake mushrooms

1 small pak choi

200g raw mixed seafood

2 tablespoons lime juice
  (1–2 limes), to taste

2 tablespoons fish sauce,
  to taste

2–3 teaspoons coconut
  palm sugar

1–2 red chillies, finely sliced

fresh coriander leaves,
  to serve

serves 2

1 Heat the coconut oil in a frying pan, add the shallots and fry over a high heat until crispy, then drain and set aside.

2 Put the stock and coconut milk in a pan with the tom yum paste, ginger, lime leaves and lemongrass. Bring to the boil, then add the mushrooms, pak choi and seafood.

3 Simmer for a couple of minutes, then season with lime juice, fish sauce and palm sugar to taste. Ladle into bowls, removing the lemongrass, sprinkle over the chillies, crispy shallots and coriander leaves and serve.

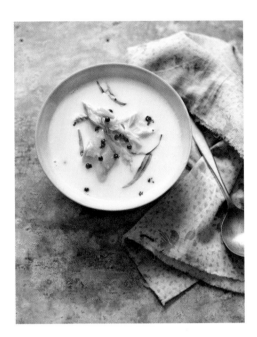

smoked haddock in coconut milk

This is a surprisingly fresh dish, despite the rich taste that often occurs in dishes using smoked fish. I vary between serving it as a soup, as it is here, and as a fish main, with a thicker sauce made by reducing the coconut liquid by a quarter once the cooked fish has been plated up.

2 smoked haddock fillets,
230g each
½ onion
2 bay leaves
2 cloves
200ml dry white wine
400ml thick coconut milk
1 tablespoon coconut oil
100g baby leaf spinach
1–2 tablespoons baby
tarragon leaves
pink peppercorns,
to garnish
sea salt

serves 2

1 Put the haddock fillets in a large frying pan with the onion half, bay leaves and cloves. Add the wine and coconut milk and poach gently until cooked, about 7 minutes. Using a large spatula, remove the fillets to a plate and cover with foil to keep warm. Skim the coconut milk liquid to remove any scum, add salt to taste, then strain through a sieve and keep it hot.

2 Melt the coconut oil in another pan and add the spinach. Cook until wilted, then drain well. Divide the wilted spinach between 2 warmed serving bowls and top with the smoked haddock, flaking it a little as you do so. Ladle the broth on top, sprinkle with tarragon and pink peppercorns, and serve immediately.

yoga bowl

This is the sort of restorative dish that your body yearns for after exercise. It is packed full of natural plant-based protein, including beta-carotine sweet potato and nutty brown rice. This is pure comfort in a bowl.

250g red lentils
2 tablespoons coconut oil
1 onion, finely chopped
4 garlic cloves, peeled and
    crushed
2.5cm piece of fresh ginger
2 teaspoons cumin seeds
1 tablespoon mild curry
    powder
1.25 litres vegetable stock
200ml thick coconut milk
250g sweet potato, peeled
    and cubed
sea salt and freshly ground
    black pepper

to serve:
coconut salsa (see page 12)
cooked brown rice

serves 4

1 Wash the lentils until the water runs clear, then drain and put in a large pan.

2 Heat the oil in a frying pan over a low heat, add the onion and sweat until soft. Add the garlic, ginger, cumin seeds and curry powder and cook for a couple of minutes to bring out their fragrance.

3 Add the onion and spices to the lentils with a pinch of salt. Cover with the stock and coconut milk. Bring to the boil and skim off any scum that rises to the surface.

4 Turn down the heat and simmer very gently, with the lid ajar, for 25–30 minutes until creamy, stirring occasionally. Add the sweet potato and cook for a further 10–15 minutes, uncovered, until the cubes are soft, but not falling apart. Add a little water if necessary, to achieve your preferred consistency, and season to taste.

5 Serve with a scoop of brown rice and a dollop of coconut salsa.

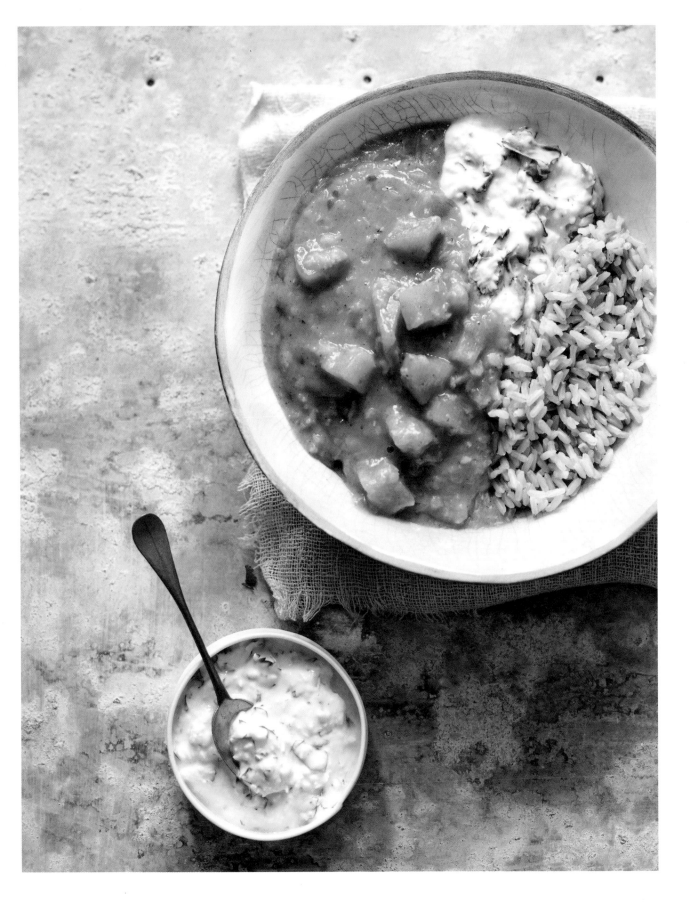

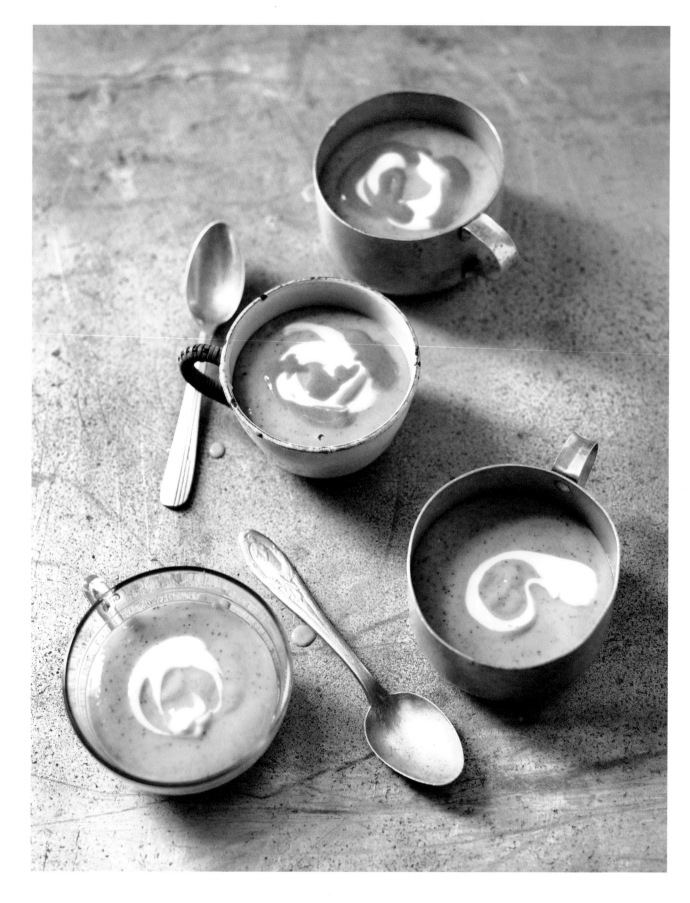

chilled avocado + yoghurt soup

Swirl a little bit of tahini here with a dollop of probiotic yoghurt. This is the ultimate naked spring time soup.

flesh of 2 large avocados,
    about 500g
3 garlic cloves
8 spring onions
3 tablespoons mint leaves
3 tablespoons coriander
    leaves
400ml vegetable stock
    (cooled)
200g plain probiotic
    yoghurt
juice of 1 lemon, to taste
sea salt and a good
    grinding of fresh
    black pepper

to serve:
tahini dressing (see
    page 16)
plain probiotic yoghurt
lemon juice

serves 4 as a starter

1 Place all the ingredients in a blender and blitz to a fine, smooth purée. Chill well. Ladle into bowls and add a swirl of tahini and yoghurt.

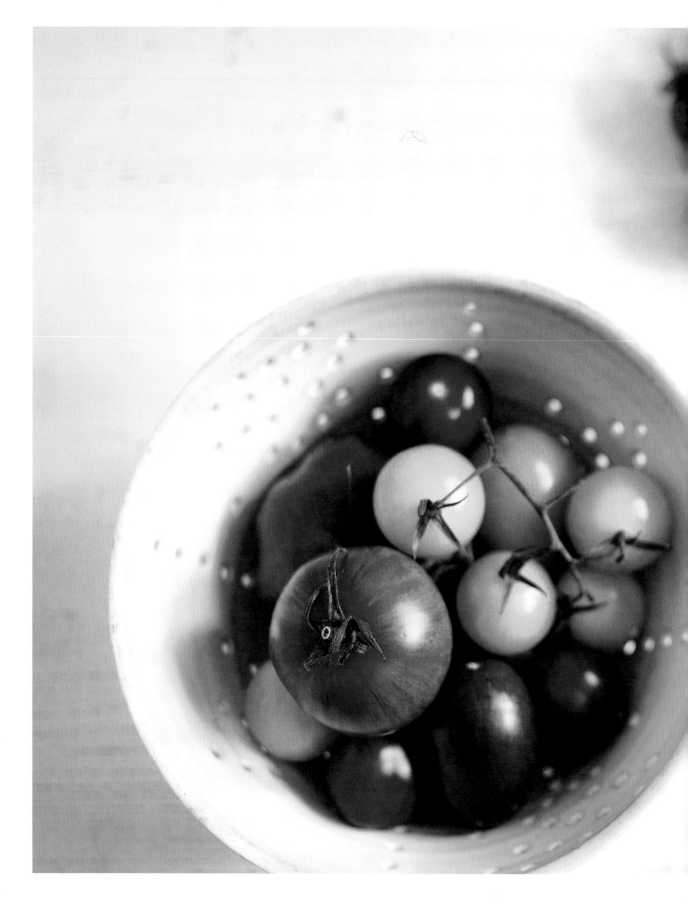

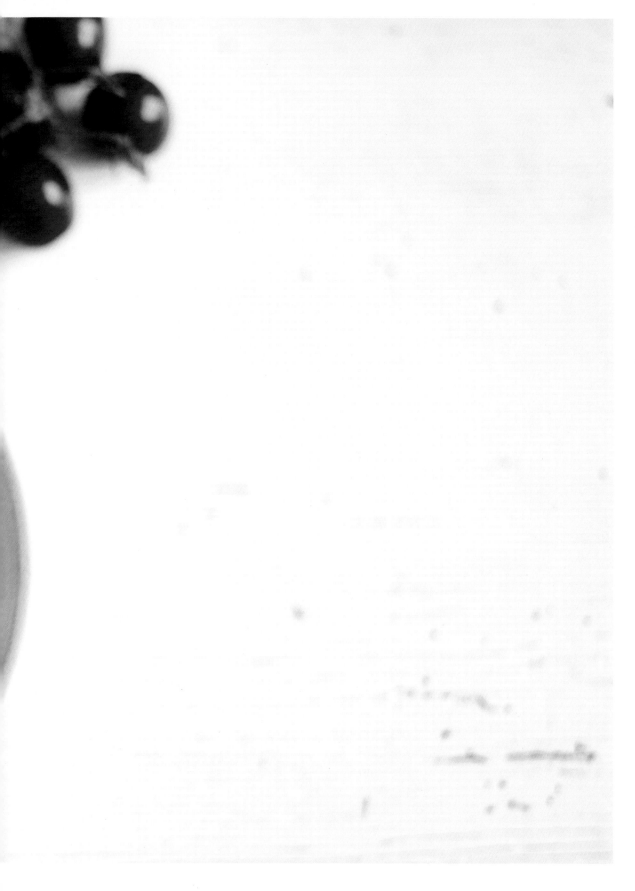

pure **raw** stripped bare nude clean detox

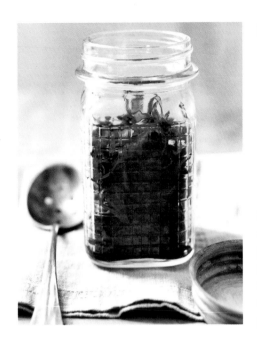

sauerkraut

Invest in intestinal bacteria today; only half an hour of work and you will have a wonderful supply of natural probiotics at your disposal for months. Made from nothing more than cabbage and salt, and any other spices and aromatics you fancy, it is a bit of a pickle to make, but worth it, as it lasts for ages. Mix it through grains and dollop onto stews.

1 medium red cabbage
**1½ tablespoons fine
  sea salt**
**1 tablespoon caraway
  seeds**

makes a 2 litre jar

1 Cut the cabbage into quarters and trim out the core. Slice each quarter down its length, making 8 wedges. Slice each wedge crossways into very thin ribbons.

2 Transfer the cabbage to a big mixing bowl and sprinkle over the salt and caraway seeds. Using your hands, work them into the cabbage by massaging and squeezing the cabbage for 10 minutes.

3 Weigh the cabbage down with a plate slightly smaller than the bowl and place a heavy object on the plate. Cover the bowl with a cloth and secure it with a rubber band or twine. This allows air to flow in and out, but not dust or insects.

4 Leave to ferment at cool room temperature (18–24°C) away from direct sunlight for 7–10 days, pressing down on the plate every so often during the first 48 hours. Check it daily and press it down if the cabbage is floating above the liquid.

5 Transfer to sterilised, dry jars and store for several months. It will keep even longer if refrigerated. As long as it still tastes and smells good to eat, it will be.

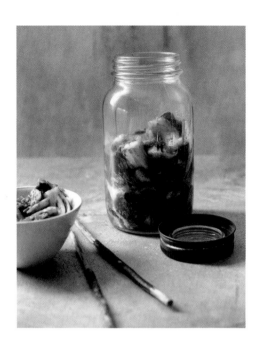

kimchi

This is a traditional spicy and sour condiment made from fermented cabbage and a variety of punchy, strong spices. It is also known for being beneficial for digestive health, and full of vitamins A, B and C. I use it alongside slippery, sesame dressed noodles or simply mixed through steamed brown rice, with some soy sauce and a fried egg.

1 large Chinese cabbage
100g coarse sea salt
4 litres water
1 head of garlic, peeled and finely chopped
5cm piece of fresh ginger, peeled and finely chopped
60ml fish sauce
60g chilli powder
1 bunch of spring onions, cut into 3cm lengths
1 teaspoon honey

makes a 2 litre jar

1 Cut the cabbage in half lengthways, then slice each half lengthways into 3 sections. Cut away the tough stem parts.

2 Dissolve the salt in the water in a very large container, then submerge the cabbage in the water. Put a plate on top to keep it submerged and leave to stand for 2 hours.

3 Mix the remaining ingredients in a very large metal or glass bowl. Drain the cabbage, rinse it, and squeeze it dry.

4 Here's the scary part: mix it all up (wear rubber gloves as the chilli can stain your hands). Pack into a clean jar large enough to hold it all and cover tightly. Leave to stand for 1–2 days at cool room temperature (18–24°C).

5 Check the kimchi: if it's bubbling a bit, it's fermenting and ready to be refrigerated. If not, let it stand another day, after which it should be ready. Once it's fermenting, serve or store in the fridge, and eat within 3 weeks.

beef carpaccio with capers + rocket

There is something unsurpassably good about the simplicity of carpaccio. The salty capers, fruity olive oil and zesty lemon combined together turn this simple, soft meat into something spectacular.

450g beef topside
big handful of rocket
4 tablespoons extra virgin
 olive oil
finely grated zest and juice
 of ½ lemon
2 tablespoons small
 capers, rinsed and
 roughly chopped
sea salt and freshly ground
 black pepper

serves 4

1 Put the beef in the freezer for 30–45 minutes. When it is firm and partly frozen, take it out and, using a very sharp knife, carefully cut into thin slices, about the width of a strand of spaghetti.

2 Place about 4 slices of beef on a large silicone baking sheet, well spaced apart. Place a second silicone sheet on top and bash with a rolling pin until the slices have expanded and thinned. You are looking to get them to about a 5mm thickness.

3 Peel off the top silicone sheet, then peel off the thin beef slices. Repeat the bashing process with the remaining slices. Season each slice with a little salt, cover in cling film and refrigerate for up to 12 hours.

4 When ready to serve, dress the rocket in a bowl with a pinch of salt and a little of the olive oil and lemon juice. Divide the beef between 4 plates, or serve on a large platter. Scatter over the capers and dress with the remaining lemon juice and zest, olive oil and a good grinding of pepper. Add a handful of rocket to each plate and serve immediately.

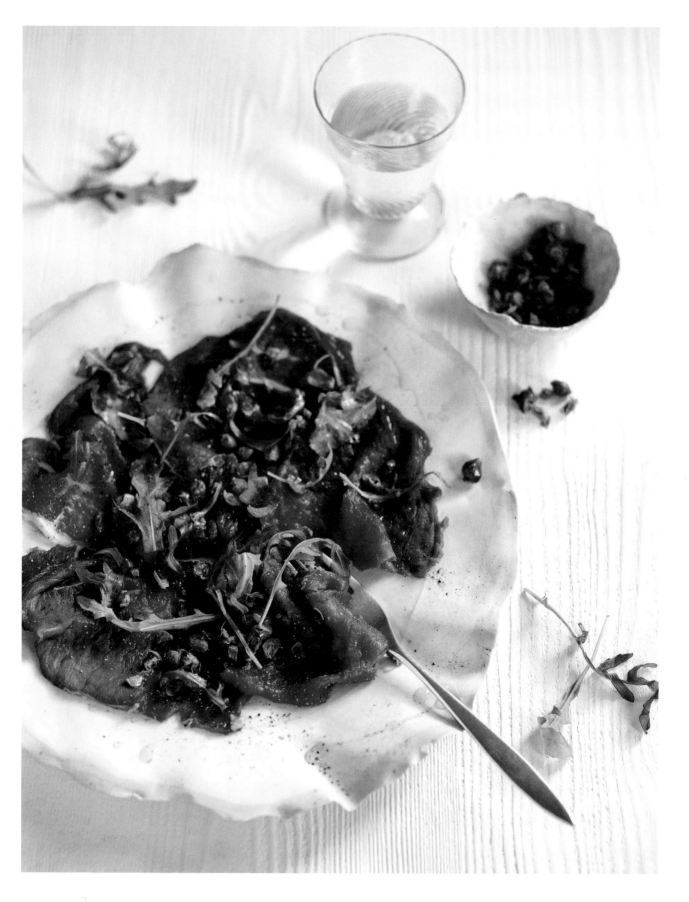

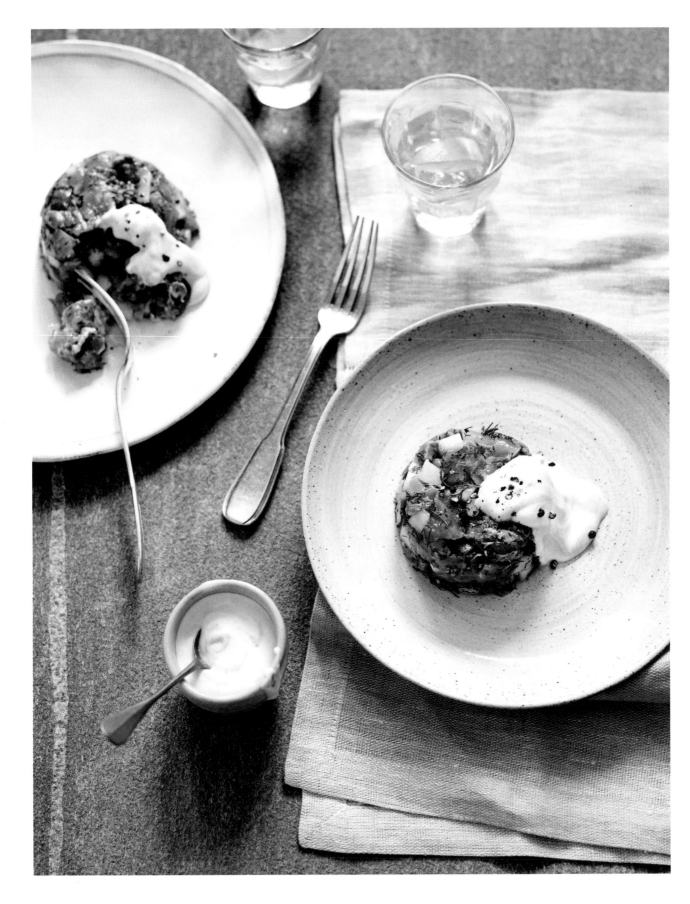

salmon tartare + wasabi crème fraîche

If eating fish raw is a new concept, then this wicked dish is a good place to start. It works as a starter, but is also great piled up in an avocado boat (see page 38). The wasabi is pretty punchy, so if it is too strong, just add another tablespoon of crème fraîche.

2 very fresh salmon fillets, about 300g in total
¼ cucumber
1 tablespoon capers, rinsed and thoroughly dried
3 heaped tablespoons dill
½ teaspoon lemon zest and 1 tablespoon juice
1 tablespoon extra virgin olive oil
good grinding of black pepper
1 quantity wasabi crème fraîche (see page 12), to serve

serves 2 as a main course, or 4 as a starter

1 If the salmon fillets have the skin on, remove and set aside, but don't throw them away (see crispy salmon skin, below). Cut the salmon into 5mm dice. Cut the cucumber into dice the same size, or a little smaller. Roughly chop the capers and dill.

2 Put the salmon in a large bowl with the chopped capers, cucumber, dill, lemon zest and juice and olive oil, and toss to combine. Press half the mixture into a greased ramekin, using the back of a spoon to compress it. Place the ramekin over a plate and invert the plate. Remove the ramekin and repeat with the remaining mixture onto a second plate. Dollop over the wasabi crème fraîche, grind over some pepper and serve.

crispy salmon skin

1 Rub a pinch of salt onto each side of the salmon skin. Heat a dry non-stick frying pan over a medium-high heat, add the skin and cook for 5 minutes on each side, or until golden and crispy. When it snaps easily, it's ready. Serve with tartare or eat it as a healthy snack.

avocado boats with pea, feta + mint

Handy for speedy meals, the pea mixture can be made in a double quantity and kept in the fridge to make this recipe even quicker. Just pop it in a lunch box with some salad leaves, grab an avocado and you have yourself a handy desk lunch.

100g frozen peas
75g feta, crumbled,
    plus extra to garnish
1 garlic clove, crushed
2 tablespoons lime juice,
    plus extra to garnish
2 tablespoons chopped
    mint leaves, plus extra
    to garnish
2 tablespoons extra virgin
    olive oil, plus extra to
    garnish
2 avocados
freshly ground black
    pepper

serves 2

1 Blitz the peas, feta, garlic, lime juice, mint and oil together in a blender. Alternatively, leave the peas to thaw and mash the ingredients together using a fork. If it's too thick, add a little more olive oil or lime juice.

2 Slice the avocados in half, remove the stones and score a few criss-cross slits into the flesh. Pile the pea purée high into each half. Add a good grinding of black pepper and a little extra feta, olive oil, lime juice and mint leaves.

dill cucumber pickle

The perfect way of eating pickled cucumber is diced and mixed with red onion and a little dill, to serve with crispy skinned mackerel, they add a powerful punch to the oily fish.

700g cucumbers, about 5–6
500ml water
500ml apple cider vinegar
3 tablespoons fine sea salt
8 dill sprigs
8 garlic cloves, peeled

makes 4 jars

1 Wash and dry the cucumbers, remove the ends and cut into thick batons.

2 Put the water, vinegar and salt in a pan and boil for 10 minutes.

3 Pack the cucumber, dill and garlic evenly into warm, sterilised jars and pour over the pickling liquid, ensuring the cucumbers are covered. Top up with water if need be.

4 Seal the jars with lids and gently tap the jars against the counter a few times to remove all the air bubbles. Store at room temperature or in the fridge. Wait at least 2–3 days before opening, to give time for the flavours to infuse. Once opened, they will last a couple of weeks in the fridge.

raw spring rolls +
peanut dipping sauce

A rainbow of colourful shredded veggies, rice paper wrappers and a mega chunky peanut dipping sauce is all it takes for these tasty spring rolls to sing. For anyone cutting out carbohydrates, I recommend steamed cabbage leaves, or lettuce leaves, instead of rice paper wrappers.

a mixture of fresh vegetables (such as peppers, radishes, cucumber, carrots, sprouted beans, celery, kohlrabi, spring onions, avocado)

6–8 rice paper wrappers (10cm rounds or larger)

1 teaspoon chopped red chilli

handful of fresh herbs, (such as mint, basil and coriander)

few edible flowers (optional, but they look pretty through the wrapper)

1 quantity chunky peanut dipping sauce (see page 15)

serves 2

1 Prepare the vegetables separately into julienne, batons or fine rounds, as appropriate. Fill a large bowl with warm water. Quickly dip in each rice paper for about 10–15 seconds, or until soft but not falling apart.

2 Place the wet rice papers on a clean surface. Arrange the prepared vegetables, chilli, herbs and flowers, if using, on each rice wrapper, about a third of the way in. Tuck in the sides and roll. The trick is to not over pack them.

3 Serve immediately with the chunky peanut dipping sauce, either whole, or cut in half for a quick bite.

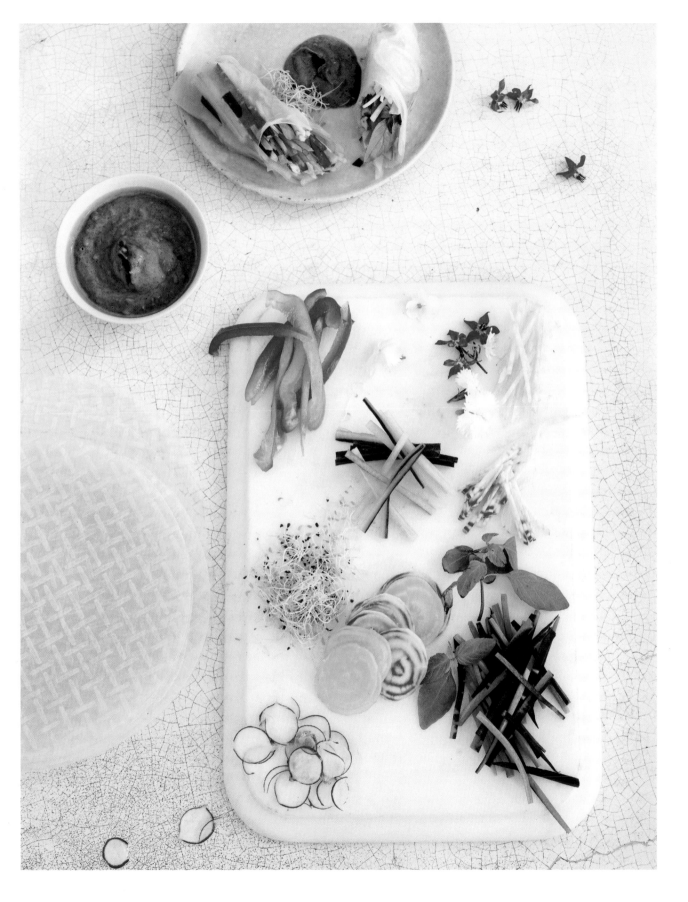

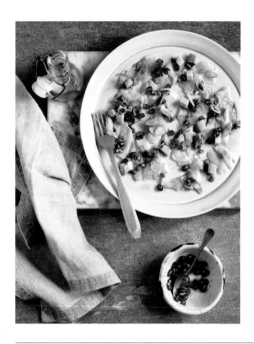

sea bass ceviche with avocado + pomegranate

Although the fish gets cold 'cooked' by the citrus juice, it is still raw, so buying fresh, sushi-grade fish is essential for ceviche. The creamy avocado works as a perfect counterpoint to the fresh pop of the pomengranate and the zesty lime-licked fish.

250g skinless, boneless
   sea bass or sea bream
   fillets
½ teaspoon sea salt
juice of 3 limes
1 green chilli, finely sliced
small handful of coriander
   leaves, roughly chopped

to garnish:
½ small avocado, diced
2–3 tablespoons
   pomegranate seeds
2 spring onions,
   finely sliced

serves 2

1 Cut the fish into thin slices and rub with the salt. Spread out in a shallow dish and leave for 1 minute, then pour over the lime juice, sprinkle over the chilli and leave to marinate for 15 minutes. If there is a lot of liquid, drain a little away, then mix through the coriander. Check the seasoning and adjust if necessary.

2 Garnish with the avocado, pomegranate seeds and spring onions.

tip
In order to get the pomegranate seeds out of their shell without too much mess, you can submerge half of it in a bowl of water before breaking it apart.

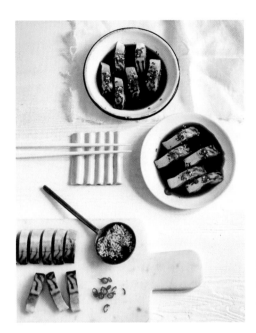

mackerel ceviche in Ponzu sauce

Ponzu is a citrusy soy sauce, which works in perfect balance with oily mackerel. Fresh, sushi-grade fish is essential for this recipe. Serve cool, but not fridge-cold, as a simple starter, or with steamed pak choi and sticky brown rice for a more substantial meal.

150g sushi-grade mackerel, filleted and pin-boned, skin on
80ml soy sauce
60ml freshly squeezed orange juice
1 tablespoon lime juice
1 tablespoon rice vinegar

to garnish:
½ red Thai chilli, thinly sliced
few fresh mint leaves, finely chopped
1–2 tablespoons toasted sesame seeds

serves 2

1 Wash and dry the mackerel gently but thoroughly. Mix the soy sauce, orange juice, lime juice and vinegar in a bowl. Strain through a sieve and set aside. Slice the mackerel into pieces 1–2cm thick.

2 If eating immediately, serve the mackerel slices sitting in a pool of Ponzu sauce with a scattering of chilli, mint and sesame seeds. If serving later, keep both the fish and sauce separately in the fridge, when ready to serve bring both to room temperature before plating.

tomatoes with capers, almonds + herbs

My all time fave salad, inspired by the colours and flavours of Istanbul. I tend to use heritage tomatoes for variation, but you could use a mixture of ripe cherry and plum tomatoes as well.

500g mixed variety
   tomatoes
3 tablespoons extra virgin
   olive oil
1 tablespoon maple syrup
1 tablespoon lemon juice
½ teaspoon smoked
   paprika
1 small shallot,
   finely chopped
2 tablespoons small
   capers, rinsed and
   roughly chopped
30g smoked almonds,
   coarsely chopped
small handful of flat-leaf
   parsley, chopped
sea salt and freshly
   ground black pepper

serves 4–6

1 Slice the tomatoes into a mixture of discs and wedges; different sizes and shapes are nice for variation.

2 Mix the olive oil, maple syrup, lemon juice and smoked paprika in a bowl and season to taste.

3 Add the shallot, capers, tomatoes, half the almonds and three quarters of the parsley. Mix together, and serve topped with the remaining parsley and almonds.

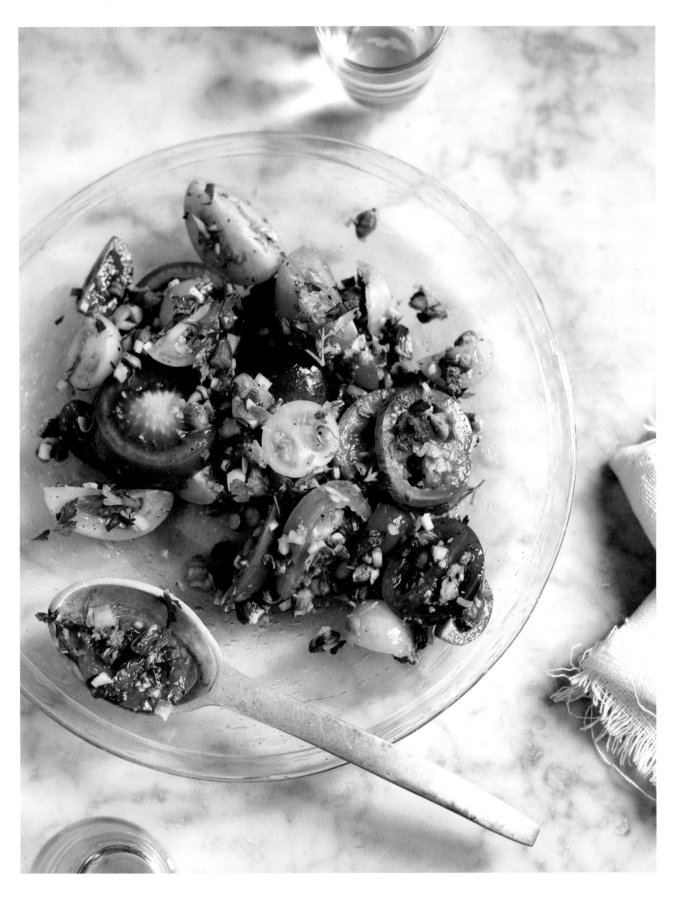

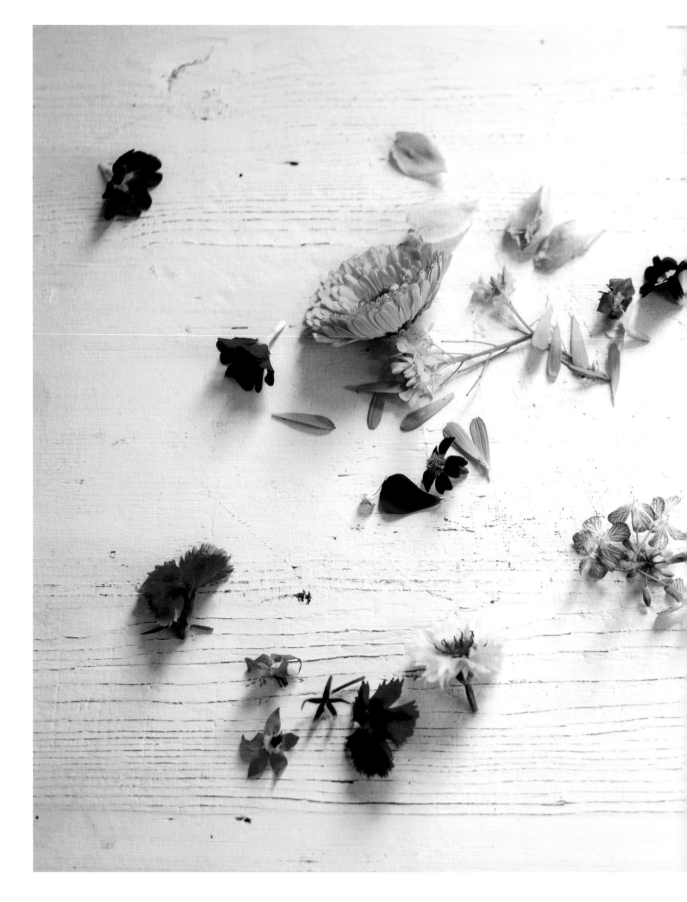

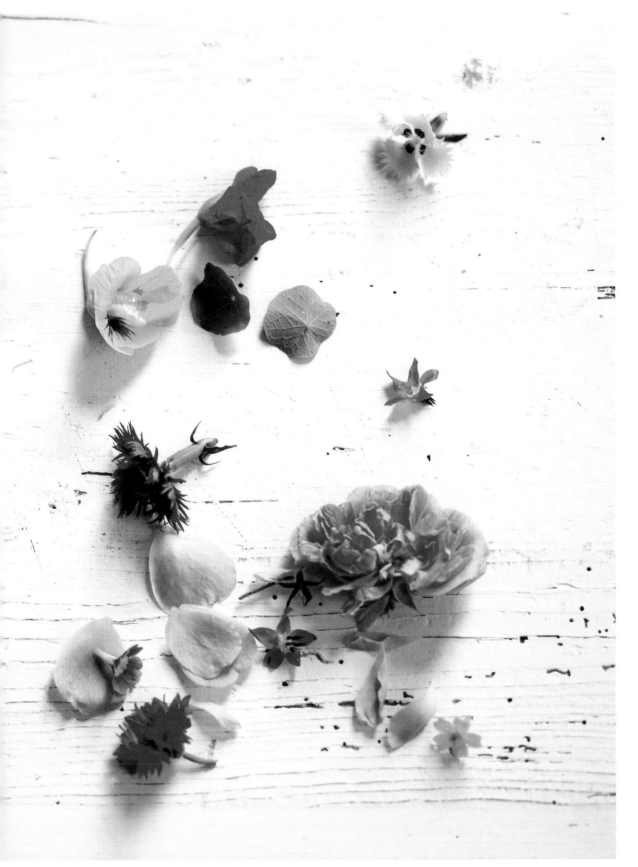

pure raw stripped bare nude clean detox

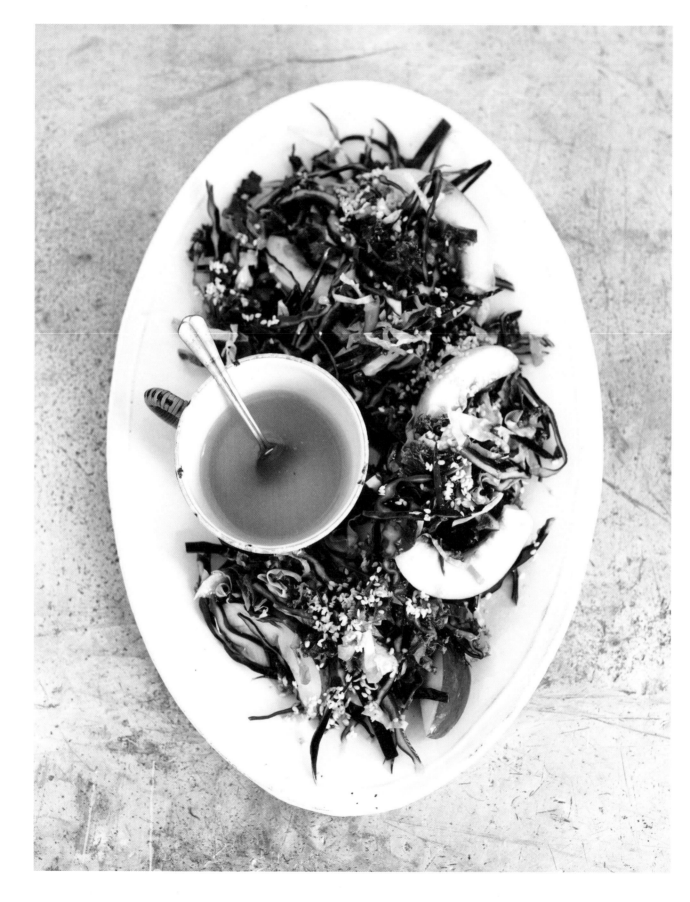

ribboned kale + nectarine salad

This is my healthy coleslaw alternative. Serve it with anything from grilled meats to other grain-based salads. Or eat it alone with a fried egg on top and a handful of toasted seeds.

150g kale

¼ small red cabbage

⅙ green sweetheart (hispi) cabbage

very large handful of chopped parsley or coriander

2 nectarines, quartered and sliced

1–2 tablespoons toasted sesame seeds

1 quantity tamari dressing (see page 17)

serves 4

1 Wash, dry and remove the stalks from the kale, then finely slice into long, thin shreds. Cut both cabbages into long thin shreds, removing the large stalks.

2 Place all the cabbage with the kale in a large steamer over a saucepan of simmering water and steam for 1–2 minutes, to soften slightly and remove bitterness, tossing them gently halfway through to ensure even steaming. Remove from the heat and plunge the kale and cabbage into a large bowl of iced water (to preserve their vibrant colour).

3 Drain and dry well and place in a large dish or platter. Add the parsley or coriander and nectarine slices and toss together gently. Sprinkle with the sesame seeds and serve with the dressing (you may not need all of it).

tip

If preparing ahead, you can dress the kale and cabbage in advance, and avoid having to steam them first; the dressing will help soften and break the kale and cabbage down, making them less fibrous.

green cauliflower 'couscous' with pumpkin seeds

This vibrant green dish is so versatile and can act as a stand-alone salad or as a rice substitute. I often swap the cheese for grilled chicken and change the broad beans for edamame or green beans.

1 head of cauliflower, stem and florets coarsely chopped
3 tablespoons extra virgin olive oil, plus extra to serve
2 garlic cloves, chopped
200g thawed frozen, or cooked fresh, broad beans
70g pumpkin seeds, lightly toasted
2 handfuls of mixed herbs, such as mint and basil, finely chopped
2 tablespoons lemon juice
100g soft goat's cheese, crumbled
sea salt and freshly ground black pepper

serves 4

1 Put the cauliflower in a food processor or blender and process to a fine couscous- or rice-like texture, in batches if you have a small food processor.

2 Heat 2 tablespoons of the olive oil in a large frying pan, add the garlic and cook until lightly golden, then add the cauliflower couscous, tossing it to coat in the garlic oil. Cook for 5 minutes, or until heated through. Transfer to a large serving bowl.

3 Add the broad beans, pumpkin seeds, herbs, lemon juice, goat's cheese and remaining olive oil. Toss until mixed. Finish with a drizzle of olive oil and season to taste. Serve warm.

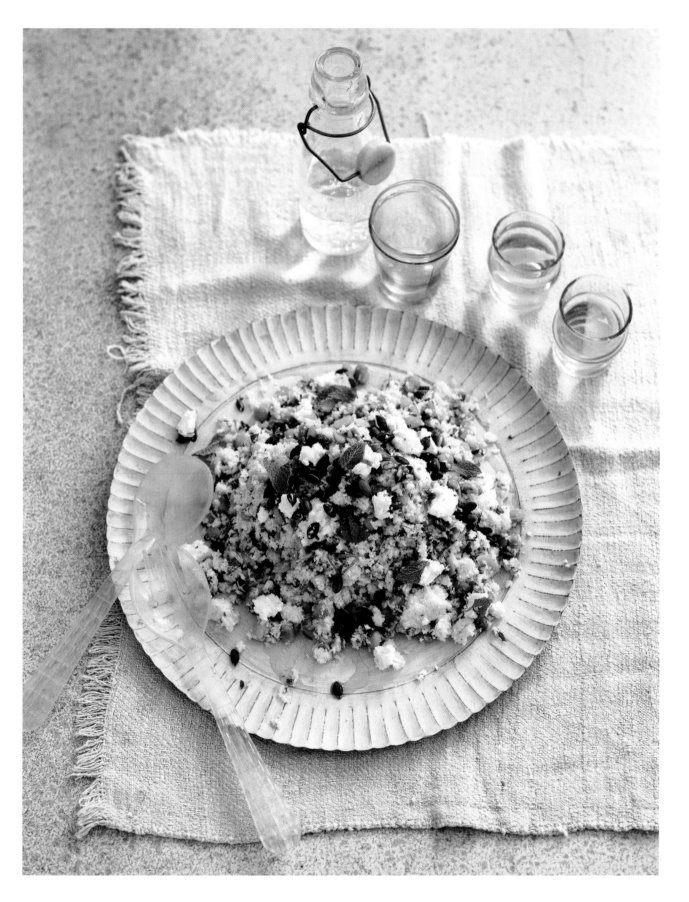

spring salad bowl

The greens I use for this vary depending on the season. In summer, it will be composed of raw salad leaves, so the steaming might only be for a few green beans or a little chard, whereas in the winter, when I feel the need for warmth, more of the greens (broccoli, cavolo nero and kale) will be steamed. The tahini dressing works superbly, although there are many other options available (see page 17).

150g garden peas
12 asparagus spears, woody ends broken off, or a handful of green beans
1 small head of broccoli, broken into florets
big handful of kale, chard or spinach
1 quantity tahini dressing (see page 17)

to serve:
1 baby gem lettuce
cress
1 tablespoon chopped chives or coriander

serves 2–4

1 Prepare a large bowl filled with ice and water and place a steamer over a pan of simmering water.

2 Steam the vegetables one type at a time, to avoid over-cooking – crunchy vegetables retain more of their goodness and are more pleasing in texture. Steam asparagus for 4–8 minutes, depending on thickness, green beans and broccoli florets for 2–4 minutes, and kale, chard or spinach for 1–2 minutes.

3 Once cooked, plunge the steamed vegetables into the icy water (this will help them retain their crispness and a vibrant green colour). If you wish to serve them hot, simply miss out this step. Serve with the tahini dressing.

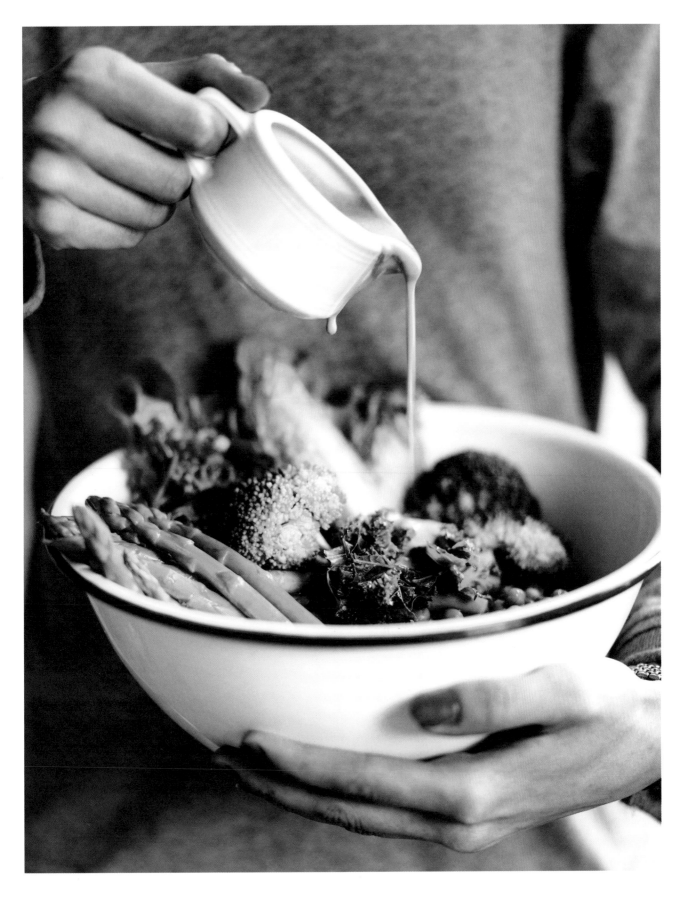

green bean, almond +
sheep's cheese salad

This quick dish is another one of of my favourite salads. The sweetness of the dried cranberries, the crunchy green beans and the salty cheese all work wonderfully together. Although this would work as a side for four, you can eat it as a main for two, with a few more handfuls of rocket, extra flaked almonds and crumbled cheese.

400g green beans, trimmed

4 tablespoons extra virgin olive oil

1–2 tablespoons lemon juice, to taste

large handful of rocket

small handful of parsley leaves

60g flaked almonds, toasted

100g sheep's cheese, crumbled

4 tablespoons chopped cranberries

sea salt and freshly ground black pepper

serves 4 as a starter, 2 as a main course

1 Bring a pan of water to the boil, add the beans and cook, covered, for 3–4 minutes, until soft to the bite but still snappable and vibrant green. Drain in a colander and run the cold tap through them until cool.

2 Meanwhile, put the olive oil and lemon juice with salt and pepper to taste in a large bowl and whisk well.

3 Add the cooled beans to the dressing with the remaining ingredients. Toss to combine, season to taste and serve.

chicory, eggs + olive salad

A light, fresh and simple dish for a speedy meal. You can also make it more substantial by serving it with cooked grains, such as spelt, pearl barley or wild rice.

2 large eggs, at room temperature
2 heads of chicory, leaves separated
60g kalamata olives, stones removed
1 quantity naked dressing (see page 17)

serves 2

1 Bring a large pan of water to the boil. When large bubbles are breaking on the surface, remove from the heat and quickly but gently lower in the eggs one at a time, using a tablespoon. Put back on the heat and boil for 6–7 minutes, depending on size.

2 Meanwhile, arrange the chicory leaves on 2 plates. Halve the olives and scatter them over each plate.

3 Drain the eggs and run cold water from the tap over them until cool enough to handle. Peel and quarter each egg and divide the quarters between the plates.

4 Drizzle a couple of tablespoons of the dressing over each and serve with a little extra salt and black pepper.

soba noodle salad with cucumber + mango

This is undoubtedly best served cold and packed up for desktop lunches or picnics. For a more substantial main, add grilled garlic prawns. They work wonders with the sweet mango and the earthy sesame dressing. For a veggie option, try it topped with a soft boiled egg; the yolk on the noodles, adds a deep, creamy richness to the dressing.

200g soba noodles
2 quantities tamari dressing
    (see page 17)
1 small cucumber, cut into
    fine strips
½ large green mango,
    cut into fine strips
4 spring onions,
    finely sliced
1 large green chilli,
    finely chopped
2 tablespoons black
    sesame seeds
small handful of coriander
    leaves, chopped

serves 4

1 Bring a large pan of water to the boil and add the soba noodles. When the water returns to the boil, add a cup of cold water and repeat this when the water comes to the boil again. Simmer vigorously for about 4–5 minutes, until the noodles are still slightly al dente. Drain and rinse well under cold water, then place in a bowl and cover with cold water to prevent them from getting sticky.

2 When ready to serve, drain the noodles and place in a bowl. Add half the dressing, the cucumber, mango, spring onions, chilli and most of the sesame seeds and coriander. Taste and adjust the dressing and seasoning.

3 Arrange on a platter or in individual bowls, top with the remaining sesame seeds and coriander and serve, with the remaining dressing.

tip
If making ahead, mix a teaspoon of olive oil into the dish to prevent the noodles from sticking and keep the dressing separate. Mix together just before eating.

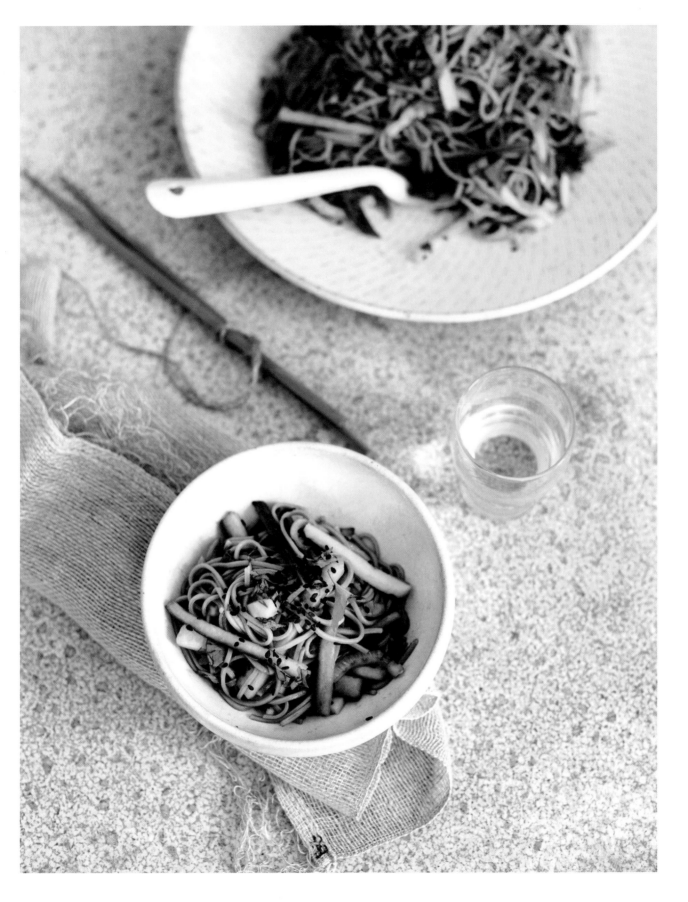

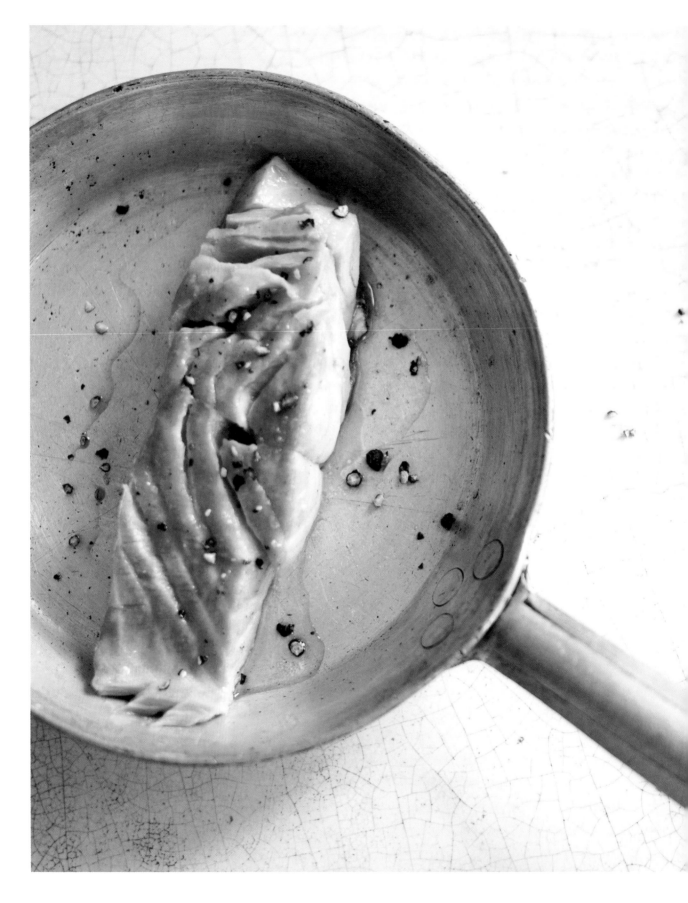

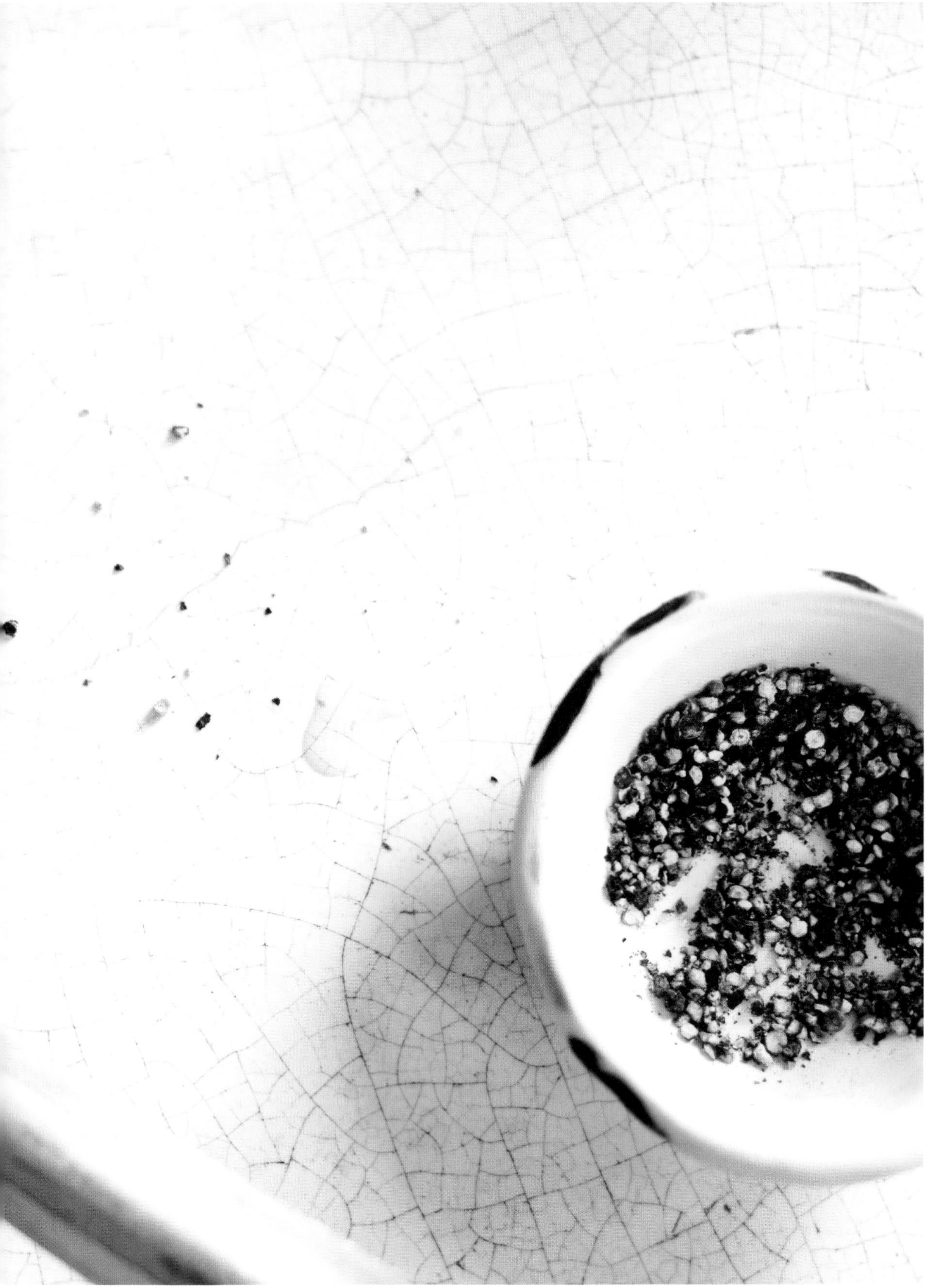

pure raw stripped **bare** nude clean detox

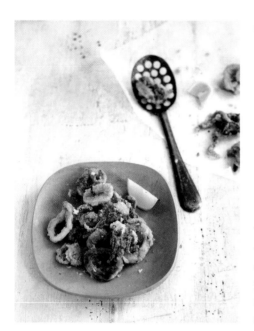

calamari with chilli, lemon + celery salt

This is an economical, no-oil-wasted recipe. It is more virtuous than your deep-fried counterpart but just as delicious, with a pleasing crunch from the semolina. If you can't find a fine semolina, just blitz a coarser one for a few seconds in a food processor. Best served with a simple salad.

500g squid, washed
    and prepared
a little milk (optional)
2 eggs
200g fine semolina
2 teaspoons chilli flakes
finely grated zest of
    4 lemons
1 heaped teaspoon
    celery salt
coconut oil, for shallow-
    frying

to serve:
lemon wedges
sea salt flakes

serves 2

1 If the squid is super-fresh, there is no need to soak it. Otherwise, soak it in some milk for 30 minutes, to tenderise it. Drain and slice into rings about 1cm thick. Trim the tentacles if you are using slightly larger squid.

2 Briefly whisk the eggs in a bowl. Put the semolina, chilli flakes, lemon zest and celery salt into another bowl.

3 Dry the squid rings thoroughly, then dip each ring into the beaten egg, then the semolina mixture, to coat. Set aside on a plate lined with kitchen paper. If you have enough semolina and egg, you can double dip them.

4 Heat a 1cm depth of oil in a deep frying pan and fry the squid in batches for 3–4 minutes, or until the crust is crisp and golden and the squid white throughout. Be careful not to over-cook or it will become tough. Top up with oil as and when you need to; the idea is to keep a little in the bottom to prevent from catching but not to swamp the pan.

5 Once each batch of calamari is cooked, transfer to another plate lined with kitchen paper, to drain any excess oil. Serve hot, with lemon wedges and sprinkled with sea salt flakes.

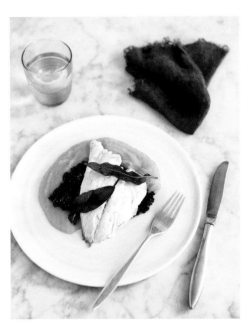

sea bass, squash + quinoa

You can use any firm white fish for this and any type of quinoa you fancy – the black just makes for a beautiful colour contrast against the delicate fish, vibrant squash purée and the sage leaves. Roasting the squash intensifies the flavour, but if you are short of time you can steam it.

½ medium butternut
squash, 250–350g, peeled
5 tablespoons coconut oil
100g black quinoa
600ml chicken or vegetable
stock
1 small onion, finely
chopped
2 garlic cloves, finely
chopped
8 large sage leaves,
4 chopped for the purée
2 sea bass fillets, or other
firm white fish
lemon juice, to taste
sea salt and freshly ground
black pepper

serves 2

1 Preheat the oven to 200°C/Gas Mark 6. Cut the squash into half moon slices and spread out on a baking tray. Drizzle with melted coconut oil, season and roast in the oven for 30–40 minutes, until golden and soft.

2 Meanwhile, toast the quinoa in a pan for 5–10 minutes, then add half the stock. Bring to the boil, then reduce the heat. Cover and cook for 15–20 minutes.

3 Heat 1 tablespoon coconut oil in a small frying pan, add the onion and sauté, then add the garlic and chopped sage. Cook for a further 2 minutes, then transfer to a blender with the squash, another 1 tablespoon coconut oil and enough of the remaining stock to blitz it to a thick paste.

4 Melt 2 tablespoons of the coconut oil in the same small frying pan until hot, and fry the whole remaining sage leaves until crispy.

5 Season the fillets and heat a large frying pan. Add 1 tablespoon coconut oil. Once hot, add the sea bass and cook over a medium heat for 2–3 minutes on each side.

6 Serve a dollop of the squash purée, top with a mound of black quinoa, then a sea bass fillet. Add a squeeze of lemon juice and a couple of fried sage leaves to each, and serve.

hainanese chicken

I was introduced to this dish by an ex-boyfriend, who used to feed it to me when I was ill. Made up of four main components – chicken, broth, cabbage and rice – it is one of the simplest and cleanest dishes. Traditionally the meal would begin with the cabbage soup and broth, with the chicken and rice for mains, but it can be eaten all together in one course too. Use white basmati as it really soaks up the flavour of the broth, but brown rice works too.

1 chicken, about 1.8–2kg
small bunch of coriander
large knob of ginger,
   whole, plus a small knob,
   chopped
2 teaspoons sea salt
1 tablespoon coconut oil
8 garlic cloves, chopped
300g basmati rice
1 small cabbage, shredded
1–2 red chillies,
   finely sliced

to serve:
soy sauce

serves 6

1 Put the chicken in a large casserole dish or pan and add enough water to cover. Separate the coriander leaves from the stalks and reserve the leaves. Tie the stalks together with string and add to the pan with the whole piece of ginger and the salt.

2 Bring to the boil, then reduce the heat, cover and simmer for 45–50 minutes, skimming off any scum or oil floating to the surface.

3 Meanwhile, heat the coconut oil in a small frying pan over a medium heat and add the chopped ginger and garlic. Fry until light golden and crispy, then set aside for the garnish.

4 Carefully remove the cooked chicken to a bowl and set aside, covered. Wash the rice in a sieve under a cold tap, then add it to the poaching liquid. Simmer for 15–20 minutes, or until cooked, adding the cabbage 3–4 minutes before the end of the cooking time. Season to taste.

5 Place the chicken on a board and shred it into large strips.

6 Serve as preferred, with the cabbage and broth, then the chicken and strained rice, with the chillies, coriander leaves and crispy ginger and garlic as garnishes. Serve with soy sauce.

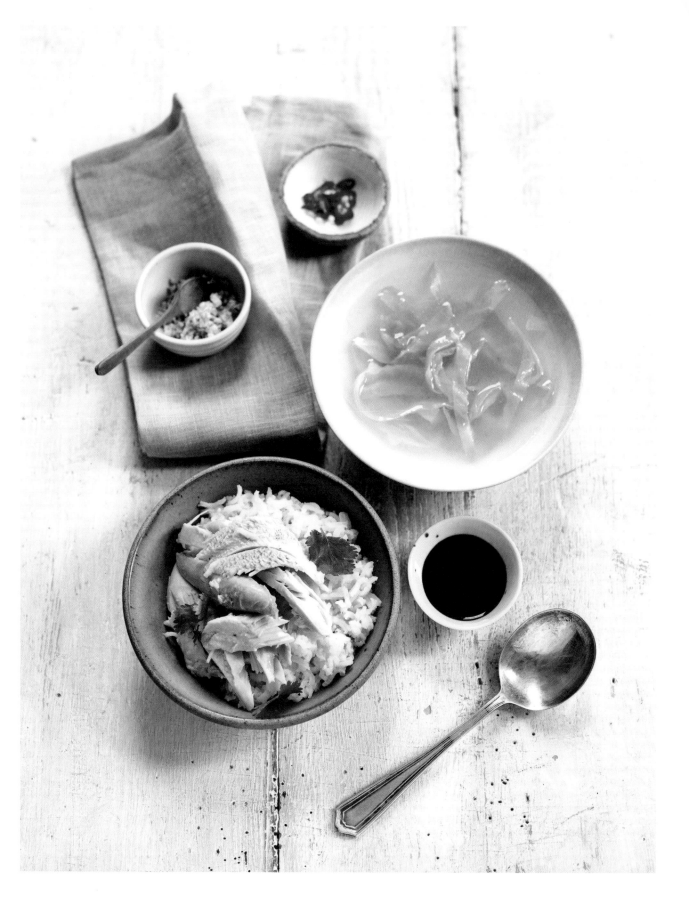

bloody Mary mussels

The spicy, smoky tomato sauce works wonders for fresh mussels. If you don't fancy making your own tomato juice, go for a shop bought brand and pimp it up or use the smoky bloody Mary recipe (without the vodka!).

1kg mussels, de-bearded and rinsed in cold water
2 tablespoons extra virgin olive oil, plus extra to drizzle
1 celery stalk, finely chopped, leaves reserved
4 garlic cloves, crushed
2 tablespoons tomato purée
500ml smoky tomato juice (see page 110) or good-quality shop bought
6 cherry tomatoes, halved and deseeded
sea salt and freshly ground black pepper

serves 4

1 Scrub and carefully check the mussels. Soak them in cold water for 20–30 minutes, to release any impurities, then drain.

2 Heat the olive oil over a medium-high heat in a large saucepan or sauté pan, wide enough so the mussels won't pile up on top of each other.

3 Add the chopped celery stalk and sweat for 5 minutes, then add the garlic and stir until fragrant, about 1 minute. Add the tomato purée and fry for a minute or two, then add the tomato juice and cherry tomatoes. Stir well and cook for another 1–2 minutes, until bubbling. Meanwhile, chop the celery leaves and set aside.

4 Add the mussels to the pan, cover and cook for 2 minutes. Check, and if they are mostly closed, continue cooking for another 2 minutes, checking every minute until they are mostly opened. Discard any that haven't opened. Taste the sauce and season, then drizzle with a little olive oil, top with celery leaves and serve hot.

miso salmon

If you can get your hands on lightly smoked salmon, it works wonders in this recipe. The smoky flavour of the fish complements the sweet and salty miso beautifully. I like to serve it with a shaved vegetable salad and tamari dressing (see page 17), or with steamed rice and kimchi (see page 33).

120ml white miso
   (fermented soybean-paste)
60ml mirin or sweet
   white wine
2 tablespoons unseasoned
   rice vinegar
2–3 tablespoons soy sauce
1½ tablespoons finely
   chopped fresh ginger
2 teaspoons toasted
   sesame oil
4 salmon fillets, 225g each
sea salt and freshly ground
   black pepper

serves 4

1 Whisk together the miso, mirin, vinegar, soy sauce, ginger and sesame oil in a small bowl. Place the salmon fillets side by side in a baking dish, pour the marinade over and turn to coat. Cover and marinate for 30–60 minutes in the fridge.

2 Heat a grill until hot. Remove the salmon from the marinade and season with salt and pepper. Place under the grill with the door open, skin side down and cook until golden brown and a crust has formed, about 3–4 minutes.

3 Turn the salmon over and cook for 3–4 minutes; you want the salmon to retain its plump pinkness in the centre. Add plenty of black pepper and serve (see introduction for serving suggestions).

lamb meatballs with rhubarb sauce

The combination of lamb and rhubarb is an unusual but delicious one. The rhubarb is laced with the heady notes of the three Cs (cardamom, cumin and cinnamon) and simmered low and slow, it turns into more of a rich spiced jam than a sauce. Pair the fragrant meatballs with brown rice, and you will have a table of happy diners.

500g lean minced lamb
1 onion, very finely chopped
2 garlic cloves, crushed
½ teaspoon cayenne pepper
1 teaspoon ground cinnamon
1 teaspoon ground cumin
1 teaspoon sea salt and
  1 teaspoon black pepper
1 small egg, beaten
1 tablespoon coconut oil

for the rhubarb sauce:
250ml chicken stock
  (see page 8)
300g rhubarb, chopped in
  8cm lengths
4 cardamom pods, crushed
4 tablespoons date syrup
½ teaspoon ground cumin
½ teaspoon ground cinnamon
200ml water

to garnish:
50g pistachios, chopped
steamed brown rice
handful of coriander leaves

1 To make the meatballs, mix the lamb mince, onion, garlic, cayenne, cinnamon, cumin, salt and pepper in a bowl, then mix in the beaten egg. Cover with cling film and rest for 30 minutes in the fridge, then shape the mixture into about 20 balls.

2 Heat the coconut oil in a large frying pan. Fry the balls in batches, about 5 at a time, until nicely browned on all sides and cooked almost through to the middle, then set aside and keep warm. Drain the fat off into a bowl.

3 Return the pan to the heat and deglaze with half of the stock. Add the rhubarb, cardamom, date syrup, spices and some salt. Add the remaining stock and the water and bring to a simmer. Cover and cook for 10 minutes until the rhubarb has broken down fully, then remove the lid and reduce the sauce until it thickens a little, about 5–10 minutes.

4 Serve the meatballs with the sauce and some steamed brown rice, the chopped pistachios and coriander leaves.

serves 4

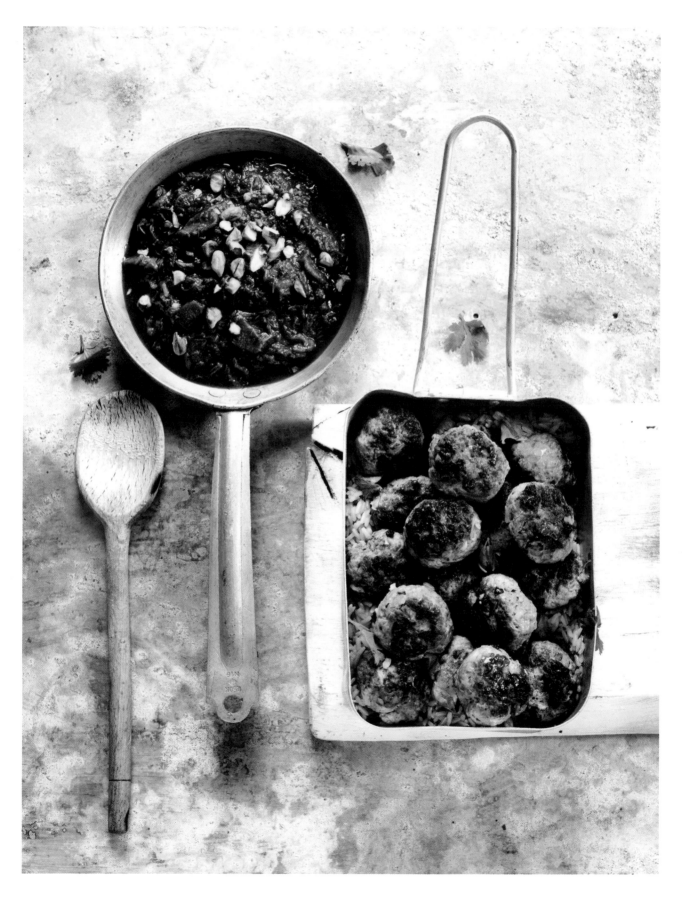

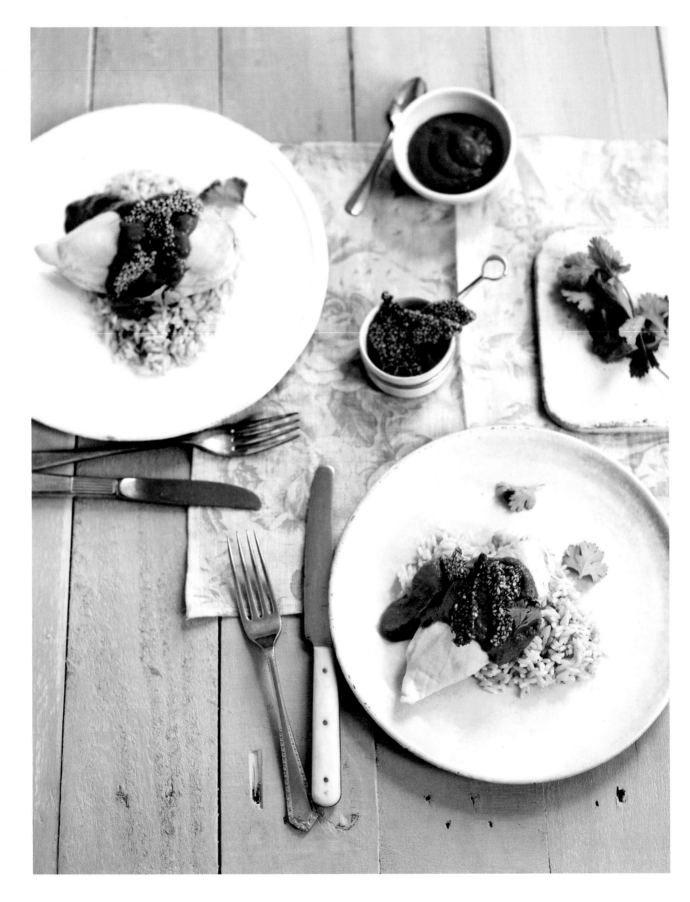

chicken breasts + red cacao sauce

Lean cuts like chicken breast call out to be paired with strong flavours. This superfood-packed sauce does just that, adding spice, depth and tomato richness to this simple meat. It is wonderful with the addition of the sesame snap, for added crunch and a little subtle sweetness.

2 large boneless,
    skinless chicken breasts
500ml chicken stock (see
    page 8)
big pinch of sea salt
handful of coriander
    leaves, to serve

for the sesame brittle:
50g sesame seeds
1 tablespoon runny honey
pinch of fine sea salt

to serve:
red cacao sauce (see
    page 15)
cooked brown rice

serves 2

1 To make the sesame brittle, preheat the oven to 180°C/ Gas Mark 4 and line a baking sheet with greased baking paper. In a bowl, mix the sesame seeds and honey together until the seeds are well coated and season. Tip the mixture onto the baking sheet and spread out in a thin, even layer.

2 Bake for 10–12 minutes, until golden brown. Take care not to over-cook. Leave to cool, then break into chunks.

3 Meanwhile, put the chicken breasts in a pan and add enough stock to cover them. Add the salt, bring to the boil over a medium-high heat, then reduce the heat to low, cover and simmer gently for 8–10 minutes. Then remove the chicken and keep warm, reserving the liquid.

4 Serve the chicken on a mound of brown rice. Spoon over some red cacao sauce and top with some sesame brittle and coriander leaves.

seared steak, cashew + goji berry lettuce cups

These asian steak cups can be served two ways, either as it is here, for starters or healthy picky finger food, or mixed together in a big salad bowl for a main course. Serve with my fresh, zesty Thai dipping sauce.

400g sirloin steaks
10–12 large baby gem
 lettuce leaves
8 radishes, finely sliced
2 spring onions, sliced
1 green chilli, finely sliced
small handful of mint and
 coriander leaves
50g roasted cashew nuts,
 roughly chopped
50g goji berries
1 quantity Thai dipping
 sauce (see page 15),
 to serve

serves 2–4

1 Heat a non-stick frying pan over a high heat, then sear the steaks for about 2–3 seconds on each side, so they are very rare. Set aside to rest for 2 minutes, then cut into thin slices.

2 Meanwhile, arrange the lettuce leaves on a serving plate. Put the radishes, spring onions, chilli, herbs, cashew nuts, goji berries and the beef into the lettuce cups. Serve with the Thai dipping sauce.

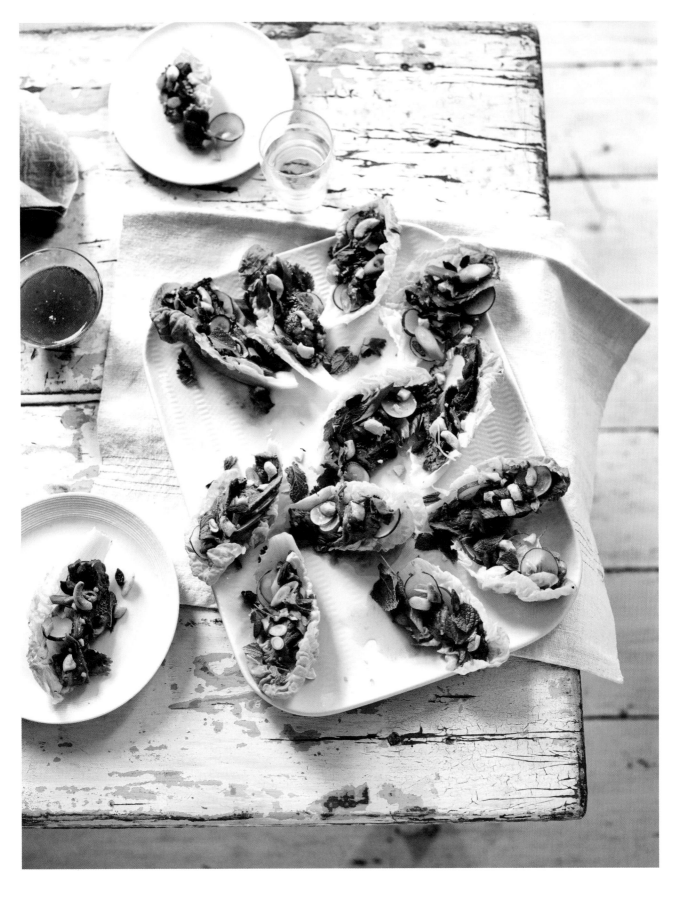

fennel + tarragon quinoa patties

As well as making wonderful little patties, this mixture also makes delicious little quinoa balls. If cooking for friends, I will often make them alongside a big bowl of leafy greens and a grain salad, but if it is just for a few people, I tend to make them smaller and serve them in large lettuce cups with slivers of avocado, ripe cherry tomatoes and lots of cucumber, radish and goat's cheese raita (see page 12).

140g quinoa
4 tablespoons coconut oil
1 onion, finely chopped
1 large fennel bulb,
    finely chopped
3 large eggs, beaten
1 teaspoon fine sea salt
15g basil leaves,
    finely chopped
15g chives, finely chopped
10g tarragon leaves,
    finely chopped
150g soft goat's cheese,
    or feta, crumbled
3 garlic cloves,
    finely chopped
about 100g fresh
    rye or spelt
    breadcrumbs

serves 4

1 Rinse the quinoa well and put in a small pan with enough cold water to cover by 2.5cm. Cook for 12–15 minutes or according to the packet instructions, then drain if necessary and set aside.

2 Meanwhile, heat 1 tablespoon of the coconut oil in a pan, add the onion and fennel and sweat over a low heat until soft and translucent, 10–15 minutes.

3 Combine the cooked quinoa, making sure it is thoroughly dry, eggs and salt in a medium bowl. Stir in the onion and fennel mixture, the basil, chives, tarragon, cheese and garlic. Stir in enough breadcrumbs to give a moist, sticky texture that holds together. Form the mixture into 12 patties or 16 ping-pong-sized balls.

4 Heat the remaining coconut oil in a large, non-stick frying pan over a medium heat and add the patties in batches (cooking too many at once means they won't turn a nice golden). Cook for 7–10 minutes on each side. If need be, increase the heat to form more of a golden crust. Remove to a plate lined with kitchen paper while you cook the remaining patties.

butternut squash pearl barley pilaf

Pearl barley makes a delicious alternative to rice in this pilaf. The combination of the squash, dates, hazelnuts and herbs adds a contrasting sweetness, nuttiness and crunch. It benefits from a squeeze of lemon and then all you need is a simple side salad to serve it with.

700g butternut squash flesh (about 1 small butternut)

4 tablespoons extra virgin olive oil

50g hazelnuts

2 garlic cloves, chopped

400g pearl barley

2 rosemary sprigs

1 litre hot chicken stock (see page 8)

80g dried pitted dates, chopped

4 spring onions, finely sliced

handful of flat-leaf parsley, chopped

sea salt and freshly ground black pepper

serves 4

1 Preheat the oven to 200°C/Gas Mark 6. Cut the butternut flesh into small chunks. Spread out on a baking tray, add half the oil and a generous grinding of salt and pepper, and toss quickly to coat. Cook in the oven for 30 minutes, tossing the squash once halfway through, until tender and the edges are starting to caramelise.

2 Spread the hazelnuts out on another baking tray and roast in the oven for about 10 minutes until golden; you will be able to smell when they are done.

3 In a large saucepan, fry the garlic for a couple of minutes in the remaining oil, until it begins to caramelise. Add the pearl barley and rosemary and stir to coat in the oil. Add the hot stock, bring to the boil, then reduce the heat and simmer for about 30 minutes, until the pearl barley is cooked.

4 Add the dates, spring onions, roasted squash and roasted hazelnuts and toss through. Keep over a low heat for a few minutes to evaporate any excess moisture. Taste and season, then stir in half the parsley.

5 Serve in bowls with the remaining parsley.

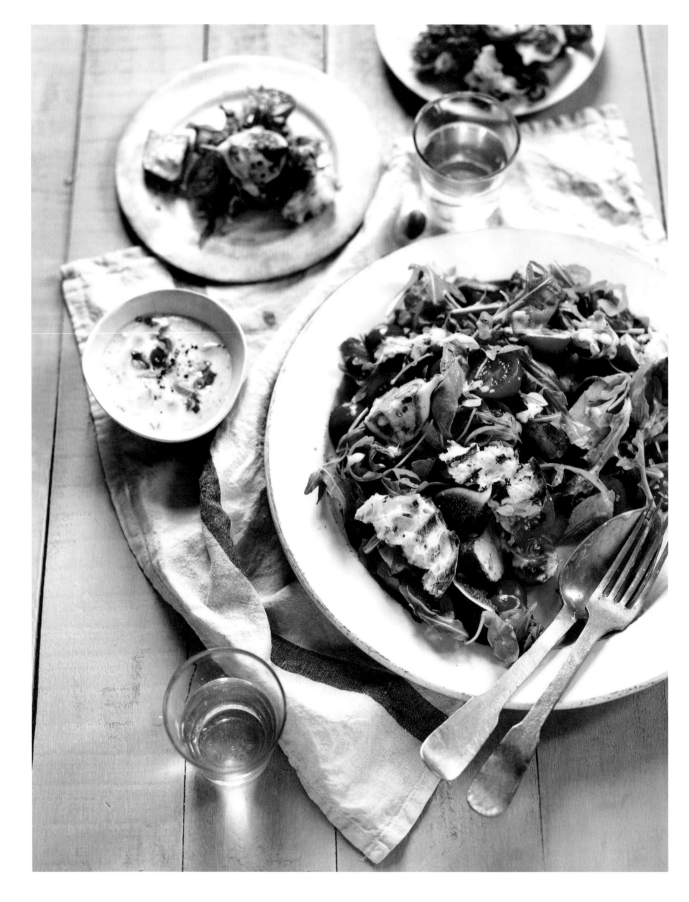

smoked tofu panzanella with figs

Tofu is certainly a bit of a crowd divider. Often thought of as an ingredient used by only hardcore vegetarians or the more culinary brave, it is an underused ingredient. I am rather impartial to most varieties, but a big fan of the smoked sort. I always buy organic, as non-organic tofu is often genetically modified.

2 slices of sourdough bread or thickly sliced gluten-free bread
large handful of rocket
small handful of basil leaves
400g cherry tomatoes, halved
200g smoked tofu, cut into 2cm slices
2 large ripe figs, quartered
1 tablespoon extra virgin olive oil
2 teaspoons apple cider vinegar
basil yoghurt dressing (see page 14)

serves 4–6

1 Heat a large griddle pan over a high heat until hot. Add your bread and place a lid on top to weigh it down. Toast until dark scorch marks appear, then flip it over and do the same on the other side. It should take 3–4 minutes on each side, but keep an eye on it.

2 Put the rocket and basil into a large bowl. Add the tomatoes, tofu and figs, then the olive oil and vinegar. Rip the charred sourdough into chunks and add to the bowl. Season with salt and black pepper and toss gently to mix.

3 Serve the panzanella with the basil yoghurt dressing drizzled on top.

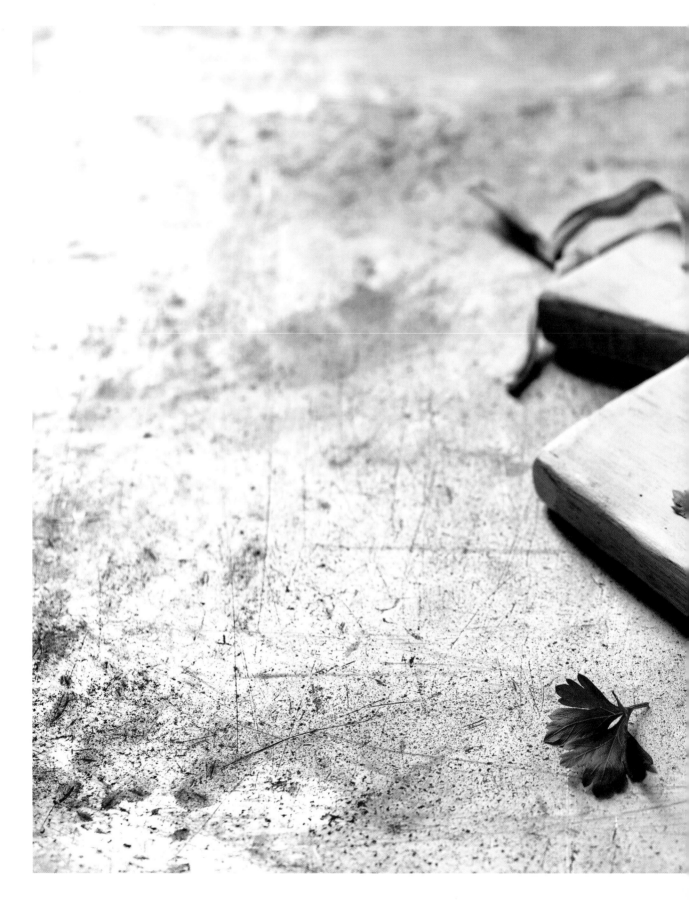

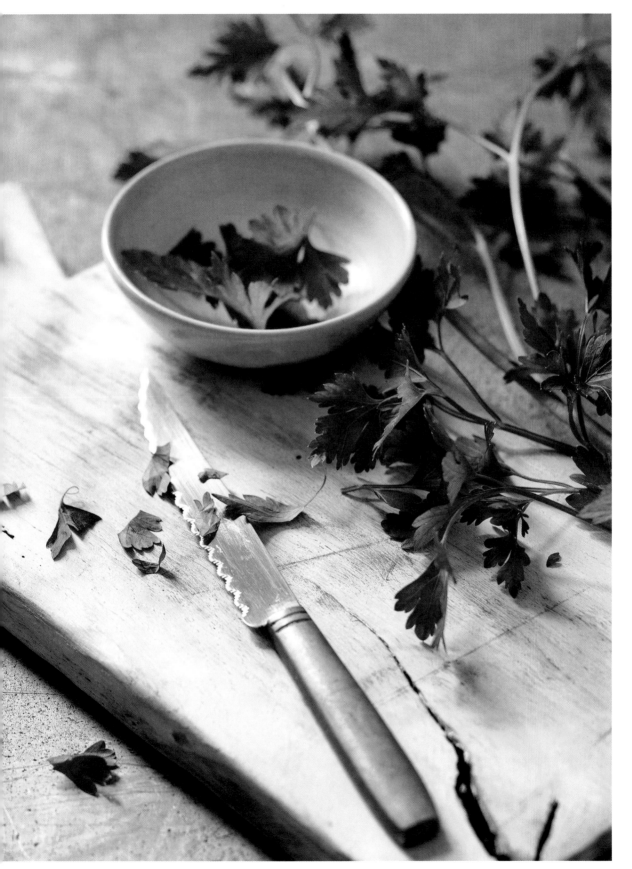

pure raw stripped bare **nude** clean detox

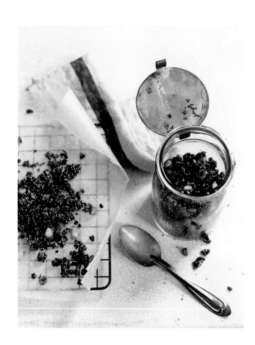

beetroot + orange quinoa granola

This nutty, crunchy granola is unlike conventional recipes. Not only is it packed full of mineral-dense beetroot, but it also has a much lower GI due to the inclusion of quinoa, which is high in protein and low in carbohydrates, and a natural sweetener called stevia (see page 119). If you use maple syrup rather than stevia, omit the orange juice and use the maple syrup as the liquid to blend the beetroot.

200g rolled oats
60g hazelnuts, roughly chopped
80g quinoa flakes
2 scant teaspoons ground cinnamon
¼ teaspoon sea salt
1 medium beetroot, 100–125g, peeled and roughly chopped
2 heaped tablespoons coconut oil
6 tablespoons date syrup or 7 large, pitted medjool dates, soaked in 60ml hot water
150ml maple syrup, or 20 drops of vanilla stevia
2 teaspoons grated orange zest and 2–3 tablespoons juice, if needed
50g goji berries

makes 1 large jar

1 Preheat the oven to 180°C/Gas Mark 4.

2 Put the oats, hazelnuts, quinoa flakes, cinnamon and salt into a large bowl. Briefly mix and set aside.

3 Put the beetroot, coconut oil, date syrup, maple syrup and orange zest into a food processor fitted with the "S" blade. Process to a sauce, adding orange juice if it seems too thick.

4 Pour the sauce over the oats and quinoa mixture and mix well. Tip onto a greased baking tray and use a spatula to smooth the mixture flat. Cook for 15 minutes, then remove from the oven and break into large pieces. Return it to the oven for a further 10 minutes, then repeat the breaking up process, stirring through the goji berries, if using. Keep cooking, turning it over every 10 minutes and breaking it up if necessary (you don't want it to be rubble), until the mixture is crunchy and golden.

5 Store in an airtight glass container for up to a week. Enjoy with nut milk, yoghurt, or sprinkled on top of smoothies.

toasted porridge with Earl Grey tea-soaked raisins

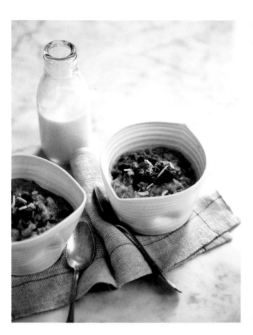

Cold days call out for warming nourishment. After too many breakfasts spent hopping around the kitchen, scalding my mouth on a half drunk cup of tea before rushing out of the door, I tried a bit of an experiment and merged my morning cuppa with my breakfast. The result: a lovely balance of creamy and zesty, the only addition needed being a few lashings of maple syrup or honey to lift the sweetness of the raisins.

50g plump raisins
1 Earl Grey tea bag
45g oats
½ teaspoon finely pared
  orange zest, plus extra
  to serve
150–200ml almond milk
½ teaspoon vanilla extract
  (optional)

to serve:
sprinkling of coconut or
  almond flakes
walnut milk
maple syrup

serves 1

1 Put the raisins and tea bag in a mug and pour over just enough boiling water to cover. Leave to soak for 10–15 minutes.

2 Put the oats and orange zest in a pan over a medium heat and toast, keeping the oats moving around the base of the pan, until they begin to release a lightly toasted aroma, about 5 minutes.

3 Remove the tea bag from the mug and set aside a few raisins for serving, then tip the contents into the oats with 150ml almond milk and the vanilla, if using. Keep stirring as soon as the porridge starts to develop little bubbles, and cook to your desired consistency, adding extra milk if needed.

4 Tip into a bowl, top with the reserved raisins, extra orange zest and flaked coconut or almonds, then serve with a little extra milk and maple syrup.

tip
You can use a chai tea bag instead of Earl Grey, and add ½ teaspoon each of ground ginger and cinnamon – warming and nourishing for winter.

gluten-free chive crêpes

I often make up a full batch of these and keep them in my fridge for quick and convenient wraps. The chives add flavour and colour, but they are also delicious plain, and are the perfect vehicle for lots of fillings.

100g buckwheat or brown rice flour
¼ teaspoon fine sea salt (optional)
250ml milk (of choice)
3 large eggs
a handful chives, finely chopped
coconut oil, for cooking

avocado + hot-smoked salmon filling:
2 large avocados
250g hot– or cold-smoked salmon, flaked
1 lemon, cut into wedges
drizzle of garlic oil (see page 10)
freshly ground black pepper

makes 6–8 (serves 2–4)

1 Mix the flour and salt, if using, in a large mixing bowl. In a separate bowl, whisk together the milk, eggs and chives. Pour this mixture into the flour mixture and stir until combined and lump-free. Let it sit for 5 minutes, then stir again and thin the mixture by adding water, a small splash at a time, until it is the consistency of double cream. (The right consistency is the key.)

2 To cook the crêpes, heat a large non-stick frying pan over a medium heat. Melt a little coconut oil and pour a scant 60ml batter to thinly coat the base, rotating the pan as you pour so that the batter runs to cover the entire base. Cook until deep golden, and the edges of the crêpe are beginning to curl and lift. Flip and brown the second side.

3 Transfer to a plate, cover with a clean tea towel and cook the remaining batter. Leftover batter keeps well in the fridge for a few days – just give it a stir and thin with a little water, if needed, before using.

avocado + hot-smoked salmon
Halve, stone, peel and thinly slice the avocados. Arrange the salmon and avocado in the centre of each crêpe, top with a squeeze of lemon, a drizzle of garlic oil (see page 10) and a grinding of pepper. Roll up and eat.

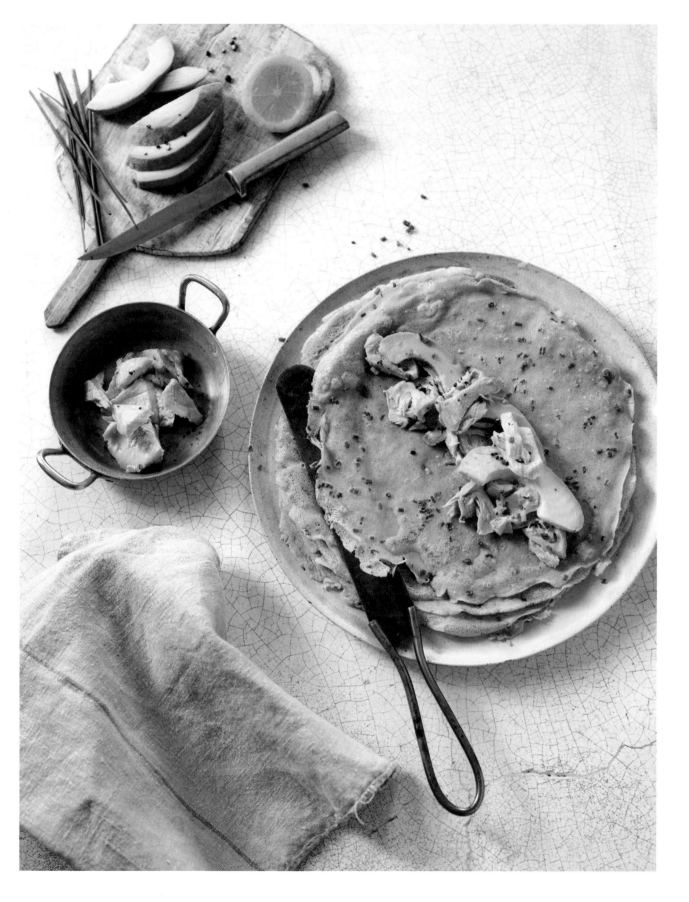

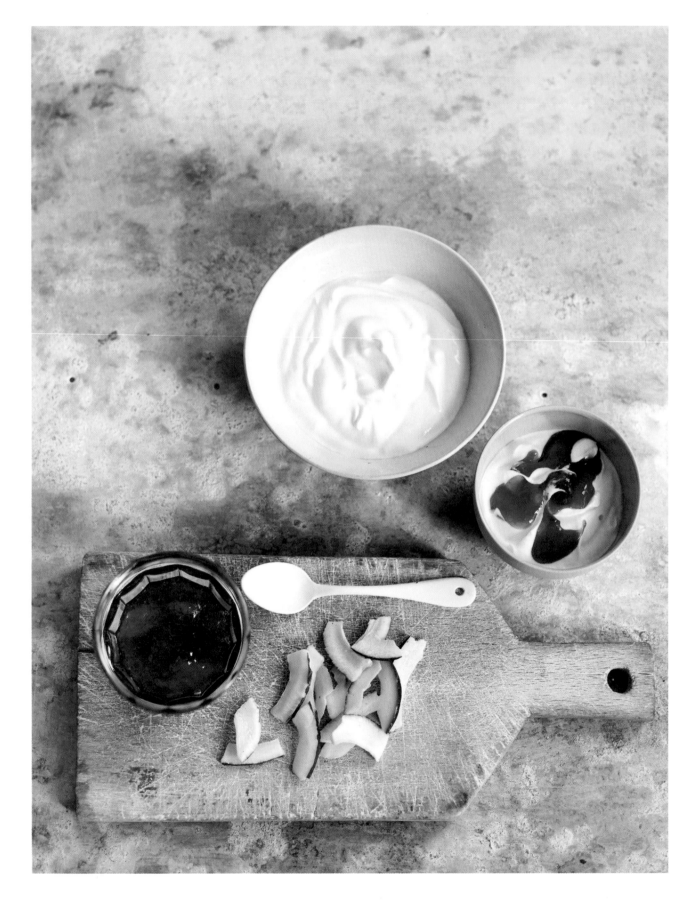

coconut yoghurt

This creamy, dairy-free yoghurt alternative is a cultured food, packed with digestive supporting probiotic enzymes. It is wonderfully smooth and creamy and lends itself well as a base. I often add spices like cinnamon, ginger and cardamom, or vanilla.

400ml tin coconut milk or 1 young green coconut
1 tablespoon fermented coconut water probiotic kefir
1 capsule (or ½ teaspoon) any probiotic to use as your starter

to serve:
small handful of flaked coconut
natural fruit compote

makes 400ml

1 Blend the thick coconut milk in a high-speed blender to achieve an even consistency. If you are using the flesh of a young coconut to make the yoghurt, add a little of the coconut water to the blender along with the flesh. Start with 100ml and add the coconut water gradually. The amount you add will depend on the thickness you want to achieve.

2 Once the coconut milk (or flesh and water) are smoothly combined, add the starter culture and give the mixture a stir through. The starter culture is what turns the coconut mixture into a yoghurt. Pour the mixture into a sealed jar and keep at room temperature for 48 hours to allow the cultures to develop and then store it in the fridge. It should last between 3–4 days.

orange blossom + thyme yoghurt
Add ½ tsp orange blossom water and 2 teaspoons honey to the coconut yoghurt.

almond + pine nut butter bars

ultimate raw chocolate coins

One of my favourite afternoon treats are flapjacks. These bars contain almond butter rather than the usual oil or butter, which makes them much higher in protein. You can use your own nut butter or buy a good-quality ready-made version, cashew and pecan butters work particularly well.

These discs of chocolate heaven are best removed from the freezer and left to thaw for just 5–10 minutes before serving (any longer and they become too soft). Toasting the nuts is the real secret, as it gives a wonderful depth of flavour. If you are not familiar with it, stevia is a plant-based sugar alternative that lifts the sweetness of the cacao. You can buy it online in liquid form or you can use 4 tablespoons coconut palm sugar in its place.

250g rolled oats
60g pine nuts
60g flaked almonds
75g chia seeds
75g dried cranberries
2 teaspoons ground cinnamon
2 teaspoons vanilla extract
150ml maple syrup or honey
170g unsalted nut butter
100g palm sugar
2 tablespoons water
big pinch of sea salt

makes 12

75g toasted pecan nuts
75g raisins
75g dates
75g toasted almonds
4 tablespoons raw cacao powder, plus
    extra for dusting, if needed
1 tablespoon coconut oil
15 drops of vanilla stevia

makes 12–14 coins

1 Preheat the oven to 180°C/Gas Mark 4. Grease a 30 x 20cm baking tin and line with baking paper.

2 Mix the oats, nuts, seeds and cranberries in a bowl. Put the rest of the ingredients in a saucepan and stir over a low heat until smooth. Add to the dry ingredients and mix.

3 Press the mixture into the tin and bake for 30 minutes, until golden. Allow to cool before cutting into bars. Store in an airtight container.

1 Blitz half the pecans with the rest of the ingredients in a food processor and chop the remaining nuts.

2 Transfer the mixture to a clean bowl and mix through the chopped pecans, then roll into a sausage shape over a sheet of cling film. If the mixture is very sticky, dust the surface with a little cacao powder.

3 Roll up to enclose, twist the ends of the cling film and place in the freezer for 30 minutes to set, then cut into discs to serve. If you leave it in the freezer for any longer, remove it 5–10 minutes before serving.

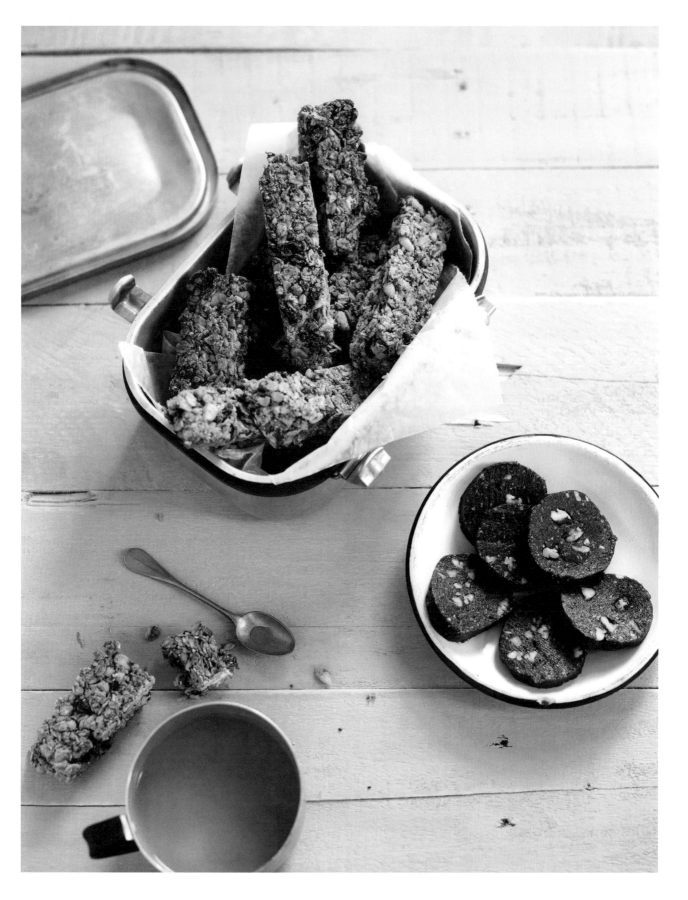

flax + pumpkin carb-free bread

It was only six months ago that this recipe first came about and it has been a staple in my kitchen ever since. No one would ever know to look at it that it is completely grain- and carb-free, so it's perfect for anyone trying to cut back on their grain intake. It is undoubtedly at its best toasted, then dolloped, drizzled and dressed with any toppings, or dips, you fancy.

250g ground flaxseed (linseed)

170g ground almonds

1 tablespoon baking powder

1 level teaspoon sea salt

70g pumpkin or sunflower seeds

5 eggs

200ml water

½ tablespoon coconut oil

makes 1 small loaf

1 Preheat the oven to 180°C/Gas Mark 4.

2 Put the flaxseed, ground almonds, baking powder, salt and three quarters of the seeds into a bowl.

3 Add the water to the dry ingredients. Beat the eggs in a large bowl until light and foamy then combine with the dry mixture. Gently stir the eggs to combine, keeping as much air in as you can, into a thick, but pourable batter. Pour into a small (500g) greased loaf tin.

4 Scatter over the remaining seeds and bake for 35–40 minutes. Turn out onto a wire rack and leave to cool before slicing and serving. It will keep for 3–4 days in a bread bin.

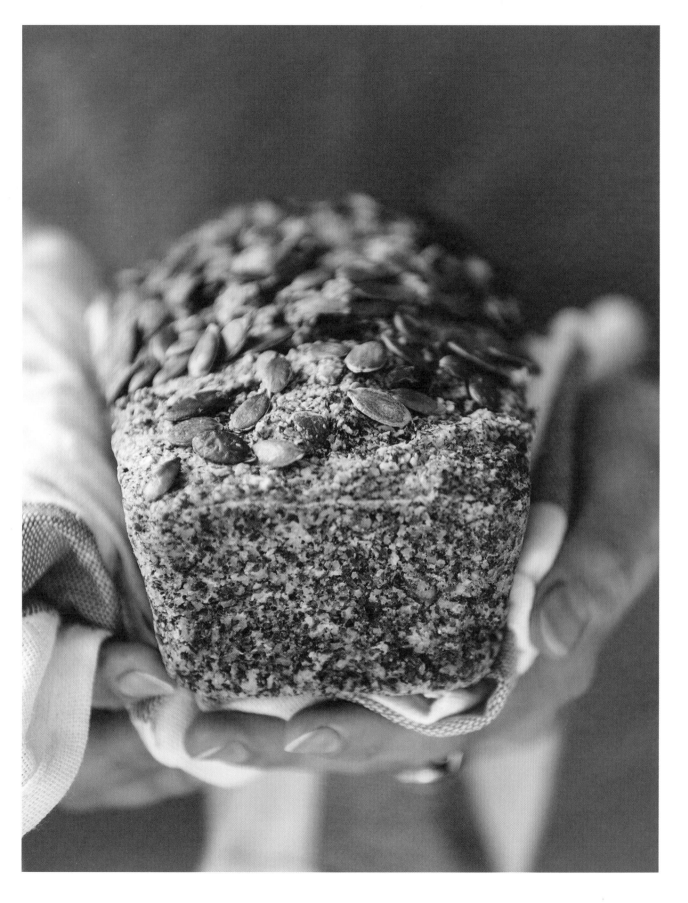

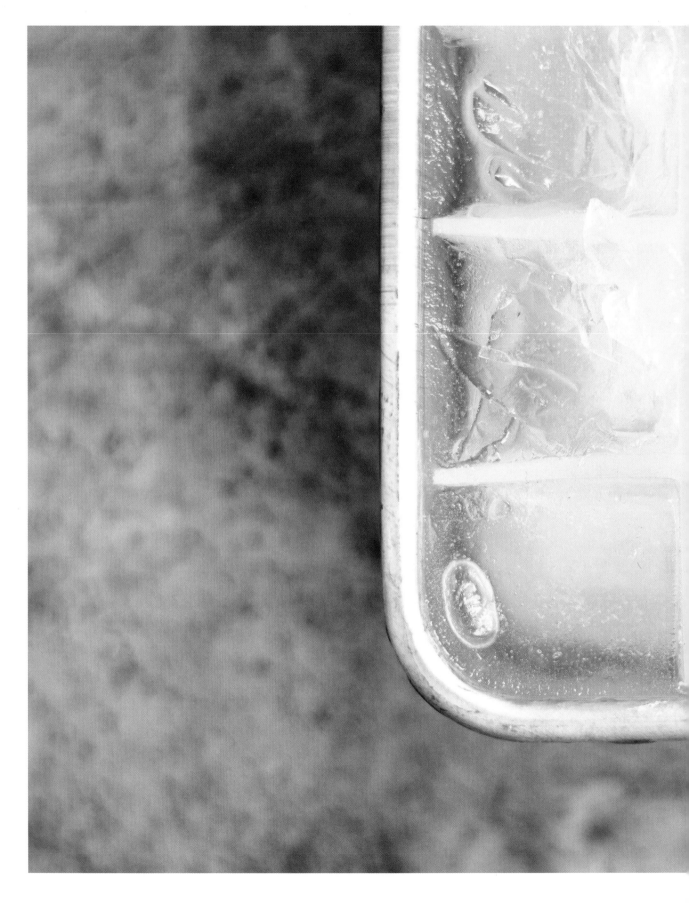

pure raw stripped bare nude clean detox

juicing

the popularity of juice

Let me ask you this: if you were to open your fridge on an average day, would you find a juice carton? I wouldn't be surprised if the answer is yes; juice is no longer considered a treat or a luxury item, but a fridge necessity, one of the staples that regularly makes their way into our shopping trolleys. The truth is that even those delicious crisp apple juices with no refined sugar, and those punchy pomegranate juices supposedly packed full of antioxidants are often no better for us than fizzy drinks. True, juices vary in quality from place to place, but even those with the revered "no added sugar" are often pasteurised, with so many of the vital vitamins and minerals removed.

what is juicing?

Juicing is a process that separates the natural liquids and fibrous structure from raw fruits and vegetables. It strips away any solid matter and leaves you with a liquid packed full of vitamins, minerals, antioxidants, anti-inflammatory compounds, and lots of phytonutrients, all ready and waiting in one convenient and hydrating drink.

the benefits of fresh juice

It might sound at this point that I am a bit of a juice sceptic, but au contraire: fresh juices are delicious and can be very beneficial, providing the body with a whole array of vitamins and minerals that are easily absorbed in the intestine because of their liquid form.

juicing diets

You may be familiar with the popularity of juicing diets, usually a 1–3 day food-less fast, where the body is fuelled by liquid alone. Despite the many declarations of their health-giving properties, I have found them to be impractical, exhausting and thoroughly uninspiring. As you can imagine, surviving on liquid alone and very little fibre doesn't fill your body with vitality and energy. Granted, they have their benefits when it comes to weight loss and vitamins but, as with all diets, they are short-lived results. If the cleanse is not carried out properly, it is easy to miss out on a lot of the beneficial fats and protein sources that the body needs to function effectively, leading to cravings and less healthy food choices once the cleanse is over. Juices are also often high in sugar which, without the fruit and vegetable fibre, enters the bloodstream rapidly and results in peaks and lows to blood sugar levels. These are just a few of the reasons why I encourage any juice-loving fanatic to approach juicing with responsibility and in conjunction with a healthy diet.

types of juicing

centrifugal Most brands you see in stores are this type of juicer.
They spin at high speed, which separates the juice from the pulp.
In terms of price and efficiency, these are the obvious choice, but
the heat generated by the blade can destroy enzymes in the fruit
and vegetables.

cold pressed/masticating The fruits or vegetables juices are
crushed and pressed hydraulically, which yields not only more juice,
but more nutrients because the juice is pressed in order to extract it.

what to juice

Of the many fruits and vegetables that can be juiced, these are my core
go-to naked ingredients. It is also possible to juice leafy greens (kale,
spinach and chard), herbs and berries too, but a lot of their goodness is
lost in the process, so I would recommend blending them instead.

fruits Lemon, lime, grapefruit, orange, kiwi, apple, pear, tomato,
pineapple, melon, watermelon, grapes

vegetables Romaine lettuce, cucumber, fennel, broccoli stalk, carrot,
beetroot, sweet potato. celery, parsnip

herbs/extras Ginger, turmeric root, chilli, parsley, coriander, mint, basil

juices

super salad juice

(pictured top right on opposite page)

This fruit-free juice is for the hardcore juicer. If it is too bitter for you, try swapping the celery for an apple.

2 celery stalks
½ cucumber
1 Romaine lettuce
a handful spinach
2.5cm piece of fresh ginger

makes 500ml

energy juice

Ginger and chilli are both natural energisers, so this is a great juice to kickstart the system in the morning.

2 large beetroot
3 oranges
2.5cm piece of fresh ginger
¼ hot chilli

makes 500ml

happiness juice

(pictured middle right on opposite page)

Pure sunshine in a glass. This also makes a wonderful smoothie if you add a few ice cubes and the flesh of a ripe young coconut.

½ large pineapple
2 apples
½ lemon
handful of mint leaves

makes 500ml

digestive juice

(pictured bottom left on opposite page)

Grapefruit works as a good cleanser, whilst the mint and fennel soothe and ease digestive enzymes.

1 cucumber
½ grapefruit
1 fennel
2 handfuls of spinach
2–4 mint sprigs
2–4 parsley sprigs

makes 500ml

cleansing juice

1 fennel bulb, including stalks
2 large cucumbers, cut into
   shorter lengths
3 handfuls of baby spinach
handful of parsley leaves
handful of mint leaves,
   with stalks

1 Put the fennel into the juicer and plunge. Put the pieces of one of the cucumbers in without plunging and fill the space around it with the baby spinach, then plunge. Do the same with the second cucumber, filling the gaps with the parsley and mint. This way the leafier greens get juiced too. Serve over ice.

makes 500ml

homemade tomato juice

3 large tomatoes, sliced
2 celery stalks, halved
½ cucumber, peeled
½ lemon, rind and pith removed
¼ hot chilli
few drops of honey or
   maple syrup (optional)
sea salt and freshly ground
   black pepper

1 Pass the tomatoes, celery, cucumber, lemon and chilli through the juicer, with salt and pepper to taste. Add the honey or maple syrup if you want to makie it a little sweeter.

2 The juice has a tendency to split, so strain it through a fine, dampened cheesecloth to remove any additional pulp if you wish.

makes 500ml

naked lemonade

(pictured bottom right on opposite page)

A natural detoxicant and energiser, this is one of my favourite cleansing juices.

5 lemons
½ teaspoon cayenne pepper
400ml coconut water
200ml filtered water

makes 500ml

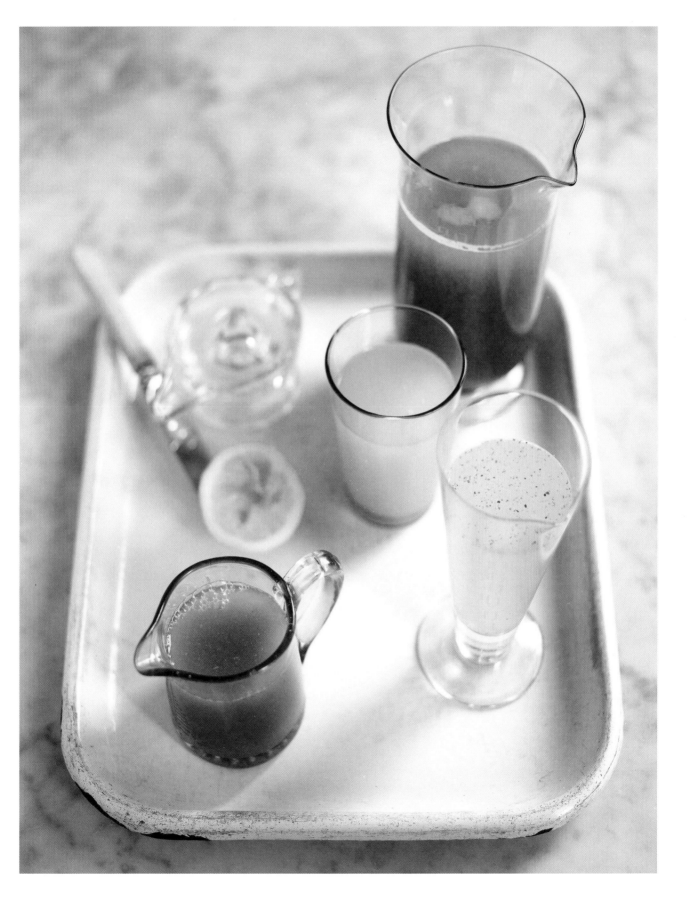

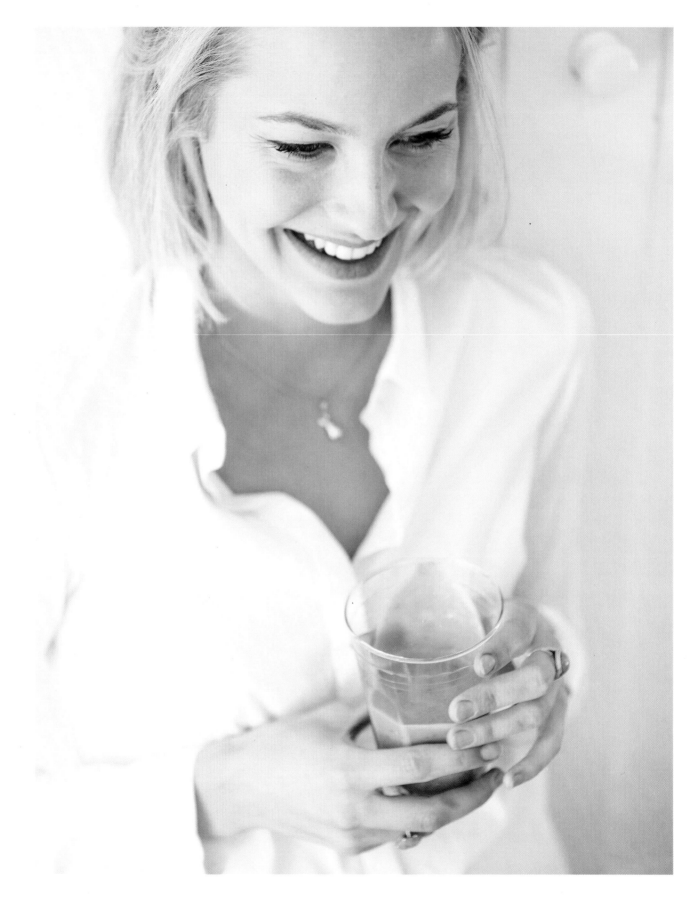

smoothies

green goddess smoothie

(pictured top middle on page 97)

This thick, creamy smoothie is packed full of mineral-dense, anti-inflammatory ingredients. It is always the one I turn to if I am run down and is my go-to if I am suffering after a night of excess. It is perfect for keeping blood sugar levels balanced. If you are on a sugar-restricted diet, replace the banana with a couple of drops of liquid stevia.

3 large handfuls of leafy greens, such as
   spinach, chard or kale
500ml water
1 avocado
½ large banana
1 heaped tablespoon chopped
   fresh ginger
juice of ½ lemon
2 tablespoons honey, or 2–3 pitted medjool dates
ice cubes (optional)
bee pollen, to serve (optional)

optional extras:
12 mint leaves (for digestion)
3–4 drops of vanilla stevia (for natural, sugar-free
   sweetness)
2 teaspoons spirulina, wheatgrass, chlorella,
   baobab or lucuma powder

1 Put all the ingredients into a blender, without the pollen if serving, and with any optional extras, and blend. You can add ice if you'd like to chill it further or to thicken slightly. Garnish with bee pollen.

serves 2

spiced banana +
pecan shake

(pictured top left on page 97)

This is a great post-workout smoothie because it contains the right mixture of protein, healthy fats and potassium the body needs for recovery. The rich toasted nuts work wonders with the warm spices and sweet toffee-tasting dates. The potassium-rich bananas are also high in amino acids, which trigger the body to produce the 'happy' hormone serotonin. Use a nut milk of your choice.

75g pecan nuts
500ml unsweetened nut milk
1 large banana, peeled, chopped and frozen
½ teaspoon ground cinnamon
½ teaspoon ground ginger
¼ teaspoon ground cloves
4 soft medjool dates, pitted

optional superfood powders:
1 teaspoon lucuma (for sweetness), maca
   (for energy), baobab (for vitamin C)

1 Preheat the oven to 180°C/Gas Mark 4. Spread the pecans out on a baking tray and roast for 15 minutes or until golden and toasted, then tip into a blender.

2 Add half the nut milk and blend until smooth. Add the remaining nut milk, the frozen banana, spices, dates and any optional superfood powders and blend.

serves 2

beetroot + cherry smoothie

(pictured bottom on opposite page)

This dark purple, cacao-laced smoothie is a pleasing combination of earthy, rich and zesty ingredients. It is filled with inflammation-fighting ingredients, like ginger and beetroot, to give your body vitamins and minerals it needs to reboot and refuel.

30g hazelnuts (or almonds or cashews)
80g frozen cherries
1cm slice of fresh ginger
250ml nut milk
1 medium beetroot, peeled and chopped
½ medium banana, frozen
1 teaspoon grated orange zest
1 heaped tablespoon raw cacao powder

optional extras:
2 tablespoons hemp protein (for a post-exercise pick me up)
small handful of oats (for a more filling breakfast smoothie)

1 Preheat the oven to 180°C/Gas Mark 4.

2 Spread the hazelnuts out on a baking tray and roast in the oven for 15 minutes, then tip into a blender. Add the remaining ingredients and blitz until smooth.

serves 2

berry + almond breakfast smoothie

(pictured middle right on opposite page)

This is best made with the addition of almond butter, but for anyone with a nut allergy you can leave this out, (instead add 2 teaspoons coconut oil). This is a great source of many vitamins and minerals and a powerful anti-inflammatory which aids digestion. It also adds a smooth creaminess. If you fancy serving the smoothie in a bowl, with superfoods or granola sprinkled on top, reduce the almond milk quantity or add another tablespoon of oats, to make it thick and spoonable.

1 banana
80g berries (blueberries and blackberries)
1–2 tablespoons oats
125ml milk (naked milk or almond milk see pages 100, 102)
1 heaped tablespoon almond butter

superfood extras:
1 tablespoon chia seeds (for omega 3)
1–2 teaspoons honey (for sweetness)
1 teaspoon lucuma (for sweetness), maca (for energy), or baobab (for vitamin C)

1 Put all the ingredients in a blender and blend until smooth.

tip
Using frozen berries and chunks of frozen banana will give you a thicker, frozen yoghurt texture which is also perfect as more of a soft-serve ice cream if you reduce the milk quantity.

serves 1

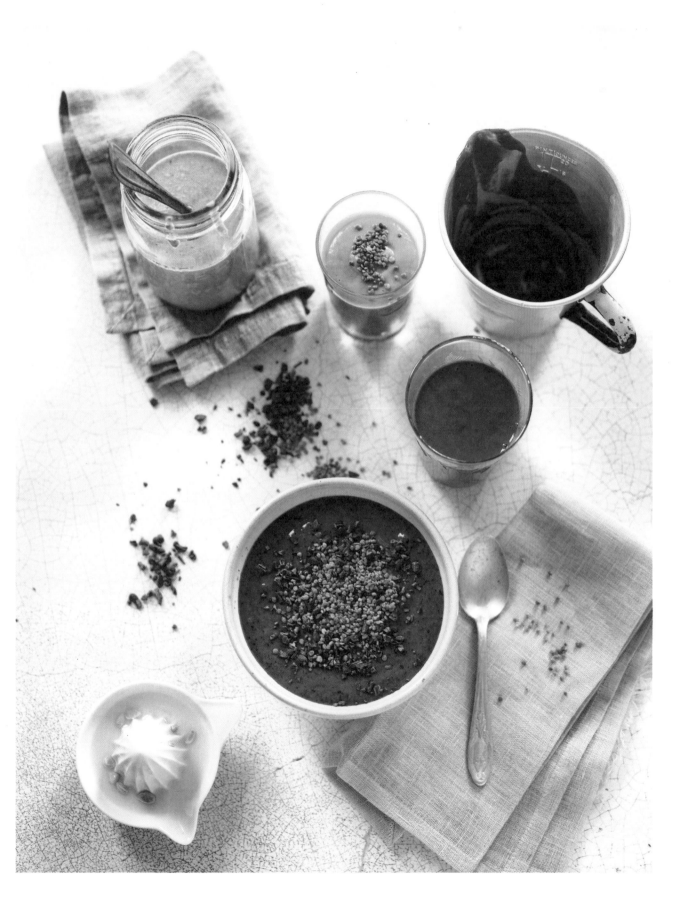

nut milks

With so many supermarkets offering a variety of different nut milks, you may wonder whether it is worth making your own. The truth is that the majority of these shop-bought products aren't as virtuous as they appear, and can contain stabilisers and emulsifiers, processed sugars and a number of unnatural flavourings or sweeteners. They are also disappointing in flavour and texture.

If you get the time, it is certainly worth making nut milks from scratch and playing around with unique combinations that no shop-bought can offer.

soaking nuts

Nuts contain small amounts of phytic acid, a naturally occurring acid that prevents them from sprouting prematurely. Although this is not strictly harmful, it contains enzyme inhibitors and can be a strain on our digestive system. Soaking nuts, before blending removes the phytic acid. Dissolve a pinch of salt in water, pour it over nuts (enough to cover them). Leave in a warm place for the specified soaking time.

roasting nuts

Roasting or heating nuts before blending them into nut milk enhances the flavour, giving the finished milk a richness and depth not found when using raw nuts. I only ever roast them myself, as pre-roasted nuts tend to be higher in naturally occurring mould. They aren't unhealthy or harmful, but they aren't as nutritious as raw or soaked nuts.

sweeteners

Opt for natural ones (see page 118) and stay away from high fructose ingredients, such as agave. My preferred choices are maple syrup, date syrup and liquid stevia. If you choose stevia, go easy on it as 1 drop is equivalent to a heaped teaspoon of sugar.

blenders

High speed blenders are certainly the best piece of kitchen kit to invest in. They achieve a smooth, velvety texture for sauces, soups, nut milks and smoothies.

However they are not cheap, and they take up space in the kitchen, so it is worth looking at other options before you commit financially.

Vitamix: Undoubtedly the best for blending liquids, like soups, smoothies and juices. The vitamix is easy to use, with a manual knob to control the speed of blend. However, it is large so requires storage space.

Magimix: This is the kit to use for larger scale blending. Making ground almonds, nut butter, grinding oats etc. Every magimix comes with three different bowl sizes, to make it convenient depending on the quantity of the recipe you are making. Like the vitamix, it is a large piece of kit so requires storage space.

Nutribullet: Portable and convenient with a sealable cup, it is the ideal blender to make single portion smoothies and cold soups. It is not as powerful as the Vitamix, so it isn't ideal for blending more fibrous green smoothies. However, it is strong enough to grind small amounts of nuts/oats into flour and making smaller amounts (approximately 1 jar) of nut butter.

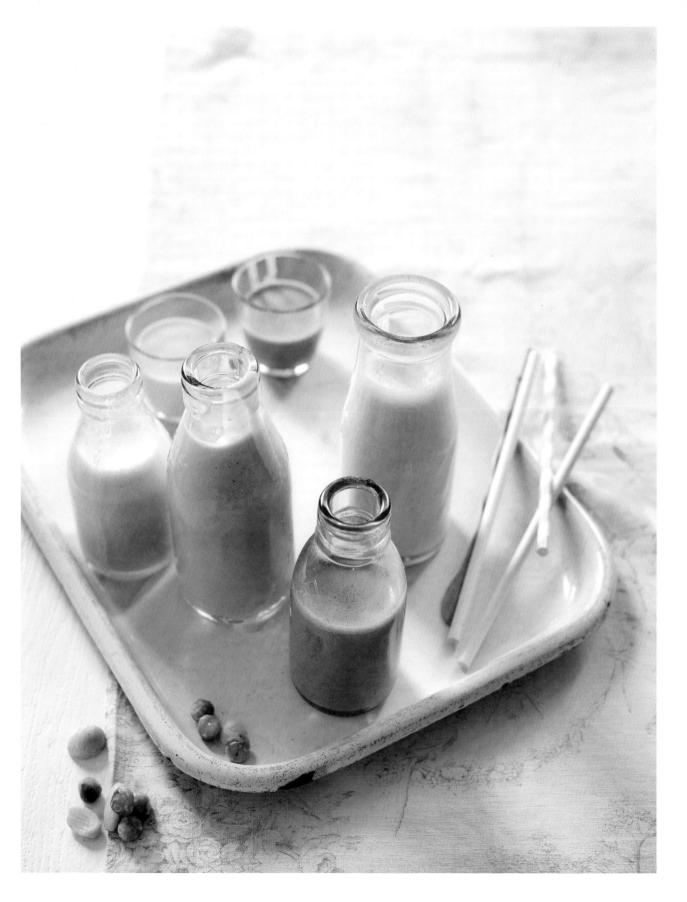

super milks

naked nut milk

(pictured middle far right on page 99)

The simplest nut milk recipe. It is a great dairy alternative to use in place of regular milk, whenever you fancy.

1 cup nuts, soaked overnight in cold water
1 litre water
1 tablespoon maple syrup
pinch of sea salt

1 Drain the nuts and discard the soaking water. Place all the ingredients in a food processor and blend on high until opaque and smooth.

2 If you want a smooth texture, pour the milk into a sieve lined with a large piece of damp muslin, set over a bowl or jug, and let it run through into the bowl. Gather the muslin around the nut mixture and twist tightly closed. Squeeze and press with your hands to extract as much milk as possible. Do this for at least 2 minutes.

3 Store in the fridge for 2–3 days.

makes 1 litre unstrained or 800ml strained

hazelnut chocolate milk

(pictured bottom far right on page 99)

This healthy chocolate milk is best used for nutshakes and iced mochas and hot chocolate.

240g hazelnuts, soaked for at least 2 hours in cold water
750ml water
4–6 tablespoons raw cacao or cocoa powder
6 tablespoons maple syrup or honey, or to taste
1 teaspoon ground cinnamon
pinch of sea salt
2 teaspoons vanilla extract

1 Preheat the oven to 180°C/ Gas Mark 4. Drain the hazelnuts, spread out on a baking tray and roast in the oven for 15 minutes, then tip into a blender.

2 Add the water and process for 2 minutes until the water has turned white and the nuts are no longer visible. Transfer the mixture to a sieve lined with a large piece of damp muslin, set over a bowl or a jug.

3 Let the milk run through the sieve into the bowl or jug beneath, then gather the muslin around the nut mixture and twist tightly closed. Squeeze and press with your hands to extract as much milk as possible. Do this for at least 2 minutes; you should get about 1 litre.

4 Rinse out the blender and pour in the filtered milk. Add the cacao or cocoa powder with your choice of sweetener, the cinnamon, salt and vanilla extract. Blend again to combine, then transfer to a jug, plastic bottle or a bowl covered with cling film, and store in the fridge for 2–3 days.

makes 1 litre

avocado milk

(pictured top left on page 99)

This nut milk is great for both savoury and sweet recipes. Blend it into smoothies, or use instead of milk in pancakes with some spinach and feta for a savoury option.

65g blanched almonds, soaked for at least 2 hours in cold water
1 litre water
½ avocado
3–4 tablespoons maple syrup
2 teaspoons vanilla extract
pinch of sea salt

1 Drain the almonds, discarding the soaking water. Rinse then put into a blender with the water and process for 2 minutes until the liquid has turned white and the nuts are no longer visible. Transfer the mixture to a sieve lined with a large piece of damp muslin, set over a bowl or a jug.

2 Let the milk run through the sieve into the bowl or jug beneath, then gather the muslin around the nut mixture and twist tightly closed. Squeeze and press with your hands to extract as much milk as possible.

3 Rinse out the blender and pour in the filtered milk. Add the avocado, maple syrup to taste, vanilla and salt and process until smooth, adding a little extra water to thin, if you like.

4 Serve cold, add to smoothies or pour over cereal. If storing, keep in a sealed jar in the fridge for up to 2 days.

makes 1 litre

macadamia + maca milk

(pictured middle far left on page 99)

The creaminess of the macadamia nuts complements the earthy taste of maca powder (the peruvian superfood) really well. Pour over granola for a omega-superfood boost.

250g macadamia nuts, soaked for 2 hours in cold water
1 litre water
4 teaspoons maca powder
1 teaspoon vanilla extract
maple syrup or sweetener of choice, to taste

1 Drain the macademia nuts, discarding the soaking water, rinse them and put into a blender with the water. Blend for 2 minutes until the water has turned white and the nuts are no longer visible.

2 Transfer the mixture to a sieve lined with a large piece of damp muslin, set over a bowl or a jug. Let the milk run through the sieve into the bowl or jug beneath, then gather the muslin around the nut mixture and twist tightly closed. Squeeze and press with your hands to extract as much milk as possible. Do this for at least 2 minutes; you should get about 500ml.

3 Rinse out the blender and pour in the filtered milk. Add the maca powder, vanilla and sweetener of choice to taste, then blend to combine. Transfer to a jug, plastic bottle or a bowl covered with cling film and store in the fridge.

makes 1 litre

sesame seed milk

The longer you soak the seeds, the better: 24–48 hours is ideal, as it activates the seeds, making them more digestible. They also blend to a creamier, smoother texture.

200g sesame seeds, soaked overnight in cold water
1 litre filtered water
small pinch of sea salt
4 drops of vanilla stevia or 2 tablespoons maple syrup and 1 teaspoon vanilla extract

1 Drain the sesame seeds, discarding the soaking water. Put into a blender with half the filtered water, the salt and stevia or syrup and vanilla and process until fully combined and smooth. Add the remaining water and blend briefly.

2 If you want a smooth texture, pour the milk into a sieve lined with a large piece of damp muslin, set over a bowl or jug, and let it run through into the bowl. Gather the muslin around the seed mixture and twist tightly closed. Squeeze and press with your hands to extract as much milk as possible. Do this for at least 2 minutes.

3 Store in the fridge for 3–4 days.

makes 1 litre

vanilla caramel milk

260g unsalted, raw
    cashew nuts, soaked for at
    least 2 hours in cold water
12 soft medjool dates, pitted
    and chopped
750ml water
2–4 tablespoons maple syrup
    and 2 teaspoons vanilla
    extract, or 4–6 drops vanilla
    stevia
pinch of sea salt

1 Drain the cashew nuts, discarding the soaking water, rinse thoroughly, then put into a blender with the dates and 850ml of the water. Blend for 2 minutes until the water has turned white and the cashews are no longer visible, adding more water if needed. Transfer the mixture to a sieve lined with a large piece of damp muslin, set over a bowl.

2 Let the milk run through the sieve into the bowl or jug beneath, then gather the muslin around the nut mixture and twist tightly closed. Squeeze and press with your hands to extract as much milk as possible.

3 Rinse out the blender and pour in the filtered milk. Add the maple syrup and vanilla, or vanilla stevia, to taste and the salt and any flavourings, if using, and blend again to combine. Transfer to a jug, plastic bottle or a bowl covered with cling film and store in the fridge for 2–3 days. Serve cold, or heat in a saucepan for a creamy hot chocolate alternative, or to add to tea or coffee.

makes 1 litre

matcha almond milk

(pictured bottom middle on page 99)

This is a straight drink rather than a base nut milk. It's a refreshing, summery alternative to café latte and is best served cold, poured over ice.

250g blanched almonds,
    soaked for at least 2 hours
    in cold water
1 litre water
2 tablespoons green tea
    matcha powder
1 teaspoon vanilla extract
maple syrup or sweetener
    of choice, to taste

1 Drain the almonds, discarding the soaking water, rinse thoroughly and put into a blender with the water. Blitz for 2 minutes, until the water has turned white and the nuts are no longer visible. Strain if desired, then add the matcha powder, vanilla and sweetener to taste. Blend until combined.

makes 1 litre

pistachio + wheatgrass milk

Blending in a quarter of an avocado (as with the avocado milk see page 101) when you add the sweetener makes this taste amazing and adds a creamy texture to the milk.

250g raw pistachio nuts,
    soaked in cold water for
    at least 4 hours
1 litre water
4 teaspoons wheatgrass
    powder
maple syrup or sweetener
    of choice, to taste

1 Drain the pistachios, discarding the soaking water, rinse and then put into a blender with the water. Blend for 2 minutes until the water has turned white and the nuts are no longer visible.

2 Transfer the mixture to a sieve lined with a large piece of damp muslin, set over a bowl or a jug. Let the milk run through the sieve into the bowl beneath, then gather the muslin around the nut mixture and twist tightly closed. Squeeze and press with your hands to extract as much milk as possible. Do this for at least 2 minutes; you should get about 1 litre.

3 Rinse out the blender and pour in the filtered milk. Add the wheatgrass powder and your sweetener of choice and blend again to combine. Transfer to a jug, plastic bottle or a bowl covered with cling film, and store in the fridge for 2–3 days.

makes 1 litre

lattes

Frothing milks takes a bit of skill. However, they can be made simpler by opting for a thicker milk. As with all lattes, an electric milk frother is the secret weapon! Also it's best to begin whisking the milk in the pan from about room temperature to ensure that you get a good volume.

chai latte

(pictured middle right on page 104)

I associate chai with my time spent in India, where it is made and drunk all across the country. I would often frequent the tiny tea stalls on roadsides, or buy a 5-rupee cup from a chai wallah on train journeys. The spices in the tea makes it delicious but they also contain a lot medicinal benefits. This spice mix quantity is a lot more than you need for this recipe, but it's worth making as it stores well in a dry place in an airtight jar, out of direct sunlight. The milk you use is completely up you. I opt for oat or almond milk.

for the chai masala mix:
50g cardamom seeds
160g black peppercorns
125g ground ginger
50g ground cinnamon
5g ground cloves
5g ground nutmeg

250ml milk (of choice)
1–2 teaspoons honey or maple syrup
1 chai tea bag

1 Grind the cardamom seeds and peppercorns together using a pestle and mortar, then mix all the spices together.

2 Put the milk, honey or maple syrup, tea bag and ⅛–¼ teaspoon chai masala mix, according to taste, into a saucepan. Place over a medium heat and, before it comes to a boil, remove from the heat and stir well. Leave to steep for 5 minutes, then remove the tea bag and heat again, until hot but not boiling.

serves 1

coffee + cacao latte

(pictured top right on page 104)

The difference between cocoa and cacao is simply in the processing: cacao is unrefined and unroasted, therefore much higher in beneficial minerals and vitamins. Whereas cocoa has been roasted at a high temperature, lowering its nutritional value and making it more bitter. Although I recommend cacao, you can also use cocoa here, reducing it to 1½ tablespoons, allowing for its extra bitterness. The milk you use is completely up you. I opt for oat or almond milk.

2 tablespoons raw cacao powder, plus a pinch
**   to serve**
200ml milk (of choice)
2 drops of vanilla stevia or 2 teaspoons
**   maple syrup**
1 espresso shot or 50ml strong filter coffee

1 Put the cacao and half the milk in a pan over a medium-low heat. As it heats up, whisk the mixture using an electric milk frother to get rid of any lumps. Once smooth, add the remaining milk and the vanilla stevia or maple syrup and continue frothing.

2 Pour espresso or filter coffee into a mug with the cacao milk, holding back the foam with a spoon. Spoon the foam over the top and add a pinch of cacao before slurping.

serves 1

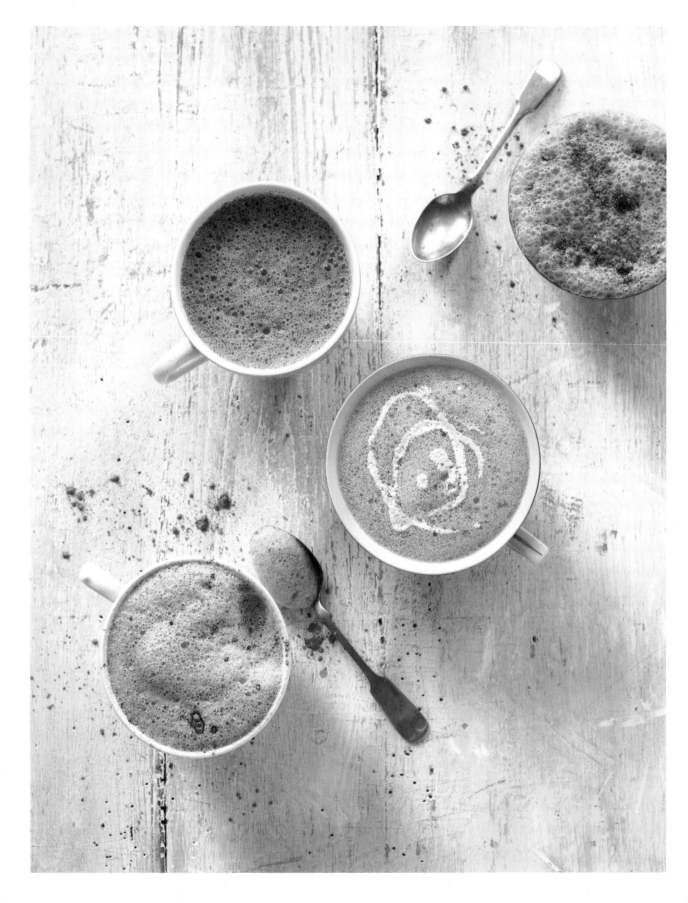

turmeric + ginger latte

(pictured middle right on opposite page)

This warming drink is one of my favourite cold-busting drinks. Although referring to it as a latte is a tad misleading as it is actually caffeine-free (which makes it a great evening tipple). To increase its medicinal benefits, feel free to swap the ground ginger for a teaspoon of freshly extracted ginger juice. The milk you use is completely up you. I opt for oat or almond milk.

1 teaspoon ground turmeric
½ teaspoon ground cinnamon
⅛ teaspoon ground ginger
250ml milk (of choice)
½ teaspoon honey, or to taste

1 Lightly toast the spices in a dry frying pan for a couple of minutes, or until they start to smell fragrant. Remove from the heat

2 Return the pan back to the heat and slowly add the milk, taking care of spluttering. Froth using an electric milk frother until bubbles form, then pour into a cup and enjoy.

serves 1

matcha + vanilla latte

(pictured bottom left on opposite page)

Matcha is a powdered green tea from Japan, made from high-grade, antioxidant-rich leaves. It makes for a wonderful latte alternative, giving a slow release of energy and providing the body with a number of beneficial vitamins and minerals. The milk you use is completely up you. I opt for oat or almond milk.

1 level teaspoon matcha green tea powder
250ml milk (of choice)
1 drop of vanilla stevia or ½ teaspoon maple
syrup, or to taste

1 Put the matcha powder in a cup and gradually add 50ml of the milk, frothing using an electric milk frother, until dissolved. Warm the remaining milk in a saucepan, whisking as it heats up and becomes light and aerated, then add the dissolved matcha. Continue frothing until hot, then sweeten to taste with vanilla stevia or maple syrup and enjoy hot, or cold over ice.

serves 1

ices

energising lemon + honey granita

(pictured left on opposite page)

This light, refreshing treat is a real favourite and acts as a great palate cleanser between courses at dinner parties. Use the best quality tea bags you can find, as it makes a great difference to the flavour.

4 green tea bags
5cm piece of fresh ginger, grated
750ml boiling water
150ml honey
6 tablespoons lemon juice

1 Put the tea bags and ginger in a medium bowl and pour over the boiling water. Cover and leave to stand for 15 minutes. Remove the tea bags and leave to cool slightly.

2 Add the honey and lemon juice and stir to combine. Strain through a sieve into a bowl and cool completely, then pour the mixture into a 20cm square baking dish, or similar. Cover and freeze for 8 hours or until firm.

3 Remove from the freezer and scrape with a fork until fluffy. Serve.

makes about 1 litre

mango + coconut ice cream

(pictured right on opposite page)

Sometimes a sorbet doesn't quite do the job. This is an alternative ice cream recipe that I came up with for one of my cooking students, who is allergic to eggs; it's creamy, rich and melts beautifully.

2 large, ripe mangos
finely grated zest and juice of 1 lemon
2.5cm piece of fresh ginger, grated
250g honey or maple syrup
500ml thick coconut milk
(use the top half of the can)

1 Peel the mangos and cut the flesh into pieces. Add to a saucepan with the lemon zest and ginger. Unless the mangos are really ripe, add a few tablespoons of water.

2 Cook over a medium heat, stirring for 10 minutes until tender. Reduce the heat and continue to cook for 15–20 minutes, until it has a jam-like consistency.

3 Remove from the heat and cool to room temperature. Transfer to a food processor, add the rest of the ingredients and process briefly; don't over-mix, as it's nice with some fruit pieces. Chill in the fridge before churning in an ice-cream machine for about 25 minutes, or according to the machine's instructions. If not serving straight away, put it in the freezer.

makes about 1 litre

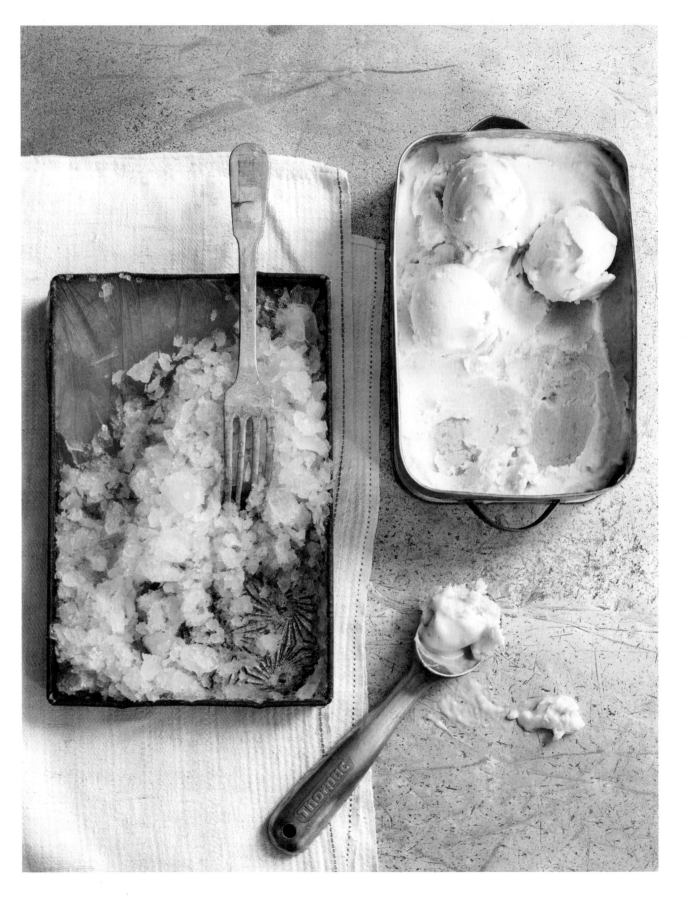

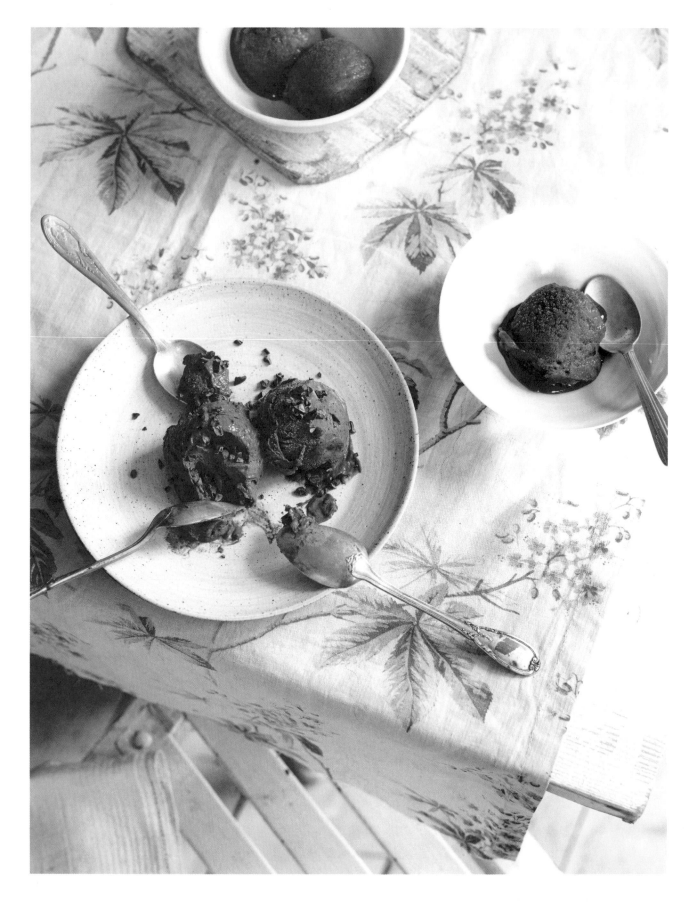

prune + bitter chocolate frozen ricotta

(pictured left on opposite page)

Rich, creamy and wickedly chocolatey, this recipe is packed full of fibre from the prunes and antioxidants from the raw cacao. It is even better if you use homemade ricotta too (see page 12).

250g ricotta
250g thick, Greek-style plain yoghurt
200g prunes, pitted and chopped
4 heaped tablespoons raw cacao powder
6 tablespoons coconut palm sugar
100g walnut halves (optional)
100ml brandy or rum (optional)
pinch of sea salt
100g raw cacao nibs, to serve

1 Put all the ingredients except the cacao nibs into a blender and blend until fully smooth.

2 Churn in an ice-cream machine for 45 minutes before transferring to a container in the freezer for a couple of hours.

3 Serve sprinkled with cacao nibs as a sticky, after-dinner dessert with a shot of coffee.

makes 1 litre

plum + Amaretto sorbet

(pictured right on opposite page)

This recipe is made in big batches in the late summer months when my mother's plum tree starts dropping its ripe wares in abundance. It's a favourite because it's so refreshingly light, sugar-free yet has a hefty kick from the Amaretto.

900g plums, stoned and sliced into eighths
300g maple syrup
1 vanilla pod
2 tablespoons Amaretto

1 Preheat the oven to 200°C/Gas Mark 6.

2 Put the plum pieces in a bowl, add the maple syrup and toss to mix. Leave to stand for 5 minutes, then transfer to a roasting tin, reserving the maple syrup liquid left behind in the bowl. Slit the vanilla pod lengthways, chop into a few pieces and add to the tin.

3 Roast for about 30 minutes until the plums are really soft and slightly blistered around the edges. Tip the contents of the roasting tin into a sieve set over a bowl and press the mixture through. Add the Amaretto and reserved maple syrup to the sieved mixture.

4 Churn the mixture in an ice-cream maker according to the machine's instructions.

serves 4–6

cocktails

smoky bloody Mary

(pictured top left and bottom right on opposite page)

This hybrid is the classic bloody Mary with a smoky twist. I have a real affinity towards this lively version, which slips down rather too easily. If you are using homemade tomato juice, be sure to add a good grinding of black pepper too.

1 litre good-quality tomato juice, chilled
1 tablespoon tomato purée
2–3 teaspoons Tabasco, or to taste
1 teaspoon Worcestershire sauce
1½ teaspoons sweet smoked paprika
1 teaspoon celery salt
1 lime, cut into wedges
300ml vodka (ideally smoked vodka)
freshly ground black pepper
celery stalks, to serve (optional)

1 In a large jug, mix together the tomato juice, purée, Tabasco, Worcestershire sauce, paprika and celery salt. Squeeze each lime, leaving some juice in each.

2 Season well and check the spice level for your taste, adjusting if necessary. Drop the lime wedges into the jug and stir together well. Cover and chill for at least 30 minutes.

3 Pour the vodka into the jug and stir well. Serve immediately, with a grinding of pepper and a stick of celery.

serves 4

lychee + mint margaritas

(pictured top right and bottom left on opposite page)

Refreshing, light and clean tasting, these are the perfect summer cocktail. If you fancy you can serve them long; especially as the addition of the coconut water is a great way to rebalance the body and keep you hydrated.

6 fresh lychees, stoned and chopped
1 mug ice cubes
250ml lime juice (10–12 limes)
80ml Triple Sec, or Cointreau
80ml tequila
coconut water (optonal, if serving long)

to serve:
lime wedges
coarse sea salt
4 mint sprigs
2 lychees, stoned and halved

1 Put all the ingredients in a blender and process until smooth.

2 Lime and salt the glass rims. Pour the mixture into the glasses and garnish with a mint sprig, lime wedge and lychee half.

3 If serving long, omit the ice from the blended ingredients and add the ice cubes to 4 glasses. Divide the blended mixture between the glasses and top up with coconut water.

serves 4

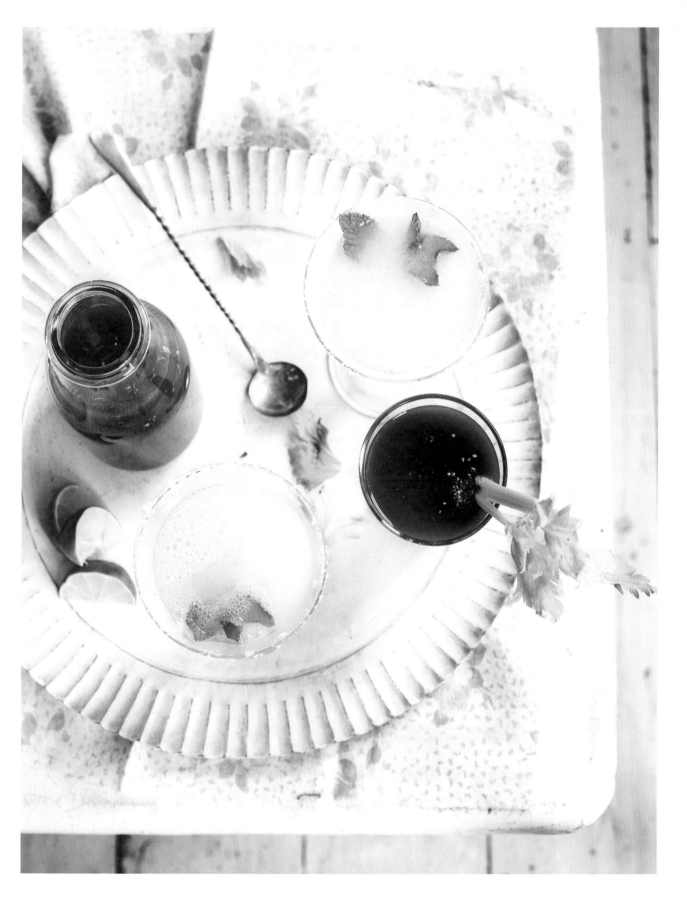

detox

why detox

Every day we are exposed to harmful toxins and chemicals, which enter the body through the air we breathe, the food we eat and the water we drink. Detoxing is about ridding the body of these built-up toxins, helping it to regenerate cells and improve overall health and vitality. True, you might say, our bodies already have an in-built system to flush these toxins out, but at times our sophisticated internal systems get overwhelmed and stop functioning at their fullest capacity.

Detoxing is all about optimising that system. It involves eating wholefoods packed with nutrients in order to boost the activity of the body's enzymes and nourish your most important detoxifying organs – the liver, lungs, kidneys, and colon – so ultimately they can do their jobs better and more efficiently.

when to detox

The time to detox is often the time you want to do it the least i.e. when you are running on low, feeling flat and unmotivated. At times like this, it is easy to turn to towards caffeine, energy drinks and sugar to keep you going but there's a more effective solution – good, old-fashioned detoxification. You may find it hard to believe that short-term dietary adjustments can be the answer to give you back lost energy, but short detoxes can help jump-start weight loss, eliminate cravings, wake up the digestive system and introduce you to a new way of eating; a mindful eating practice.

how to detox

A major component of any detox or cleanse is a healthy diet. Why? Detoxification programmes that combine short-term dietary changes with nourishing foods that support the liver's detoxification enzyme systems have been shown to significantly reduce tiredness, pain and other symptoms in patients with chronic fatigue syndrome, fibromyalgia and other chronic conditions. The dietary component of a detox-cleanse typically involves making short-term dietary adjustments that are designed to accomplish a number of objectives.

You can detox easily and effectively whilst you continue to eat, as long as you are cutting out the foods and substances that interfere with the detoxification process. Processed foods should be avoided – nothing from a box, jar or can. You want to only eat fresh food (organic, if possible) starting with 3 days and, if strong, going up to 10.

digestion detox

what is the digestion detox?

The digestive system is the gateway to the body, the interface and protective barrier between you and the outside world. It acts like a skin on the inside, keeping out the bad stuff and letting the good stuff in, taking in food, breaking it down and turning it into a liquid form through which we can absorb its nutrients.

We have an amazing digestive system that allows for a range of different types of foods to be processed, and our body's ability to do this is crucial to our overall health. An impaired system can be detrimental to not only our energy but also our mood, immunity and quality of life. In its most simple terms, we should all be aware just how effectively our body processes and absorbs the nutrients from the food and drinks we consume, because there is nothing more important than having a fully functioning digestive system.

The quality and nutritional properties of the food we eat plays a vital role in maintaining the balance of bacteria in the digestive tract. Having a balanced gut flora is crucial to its ability to process foods. The increase in pre-packaged, convenience and highly processed foods can largely be blamed for the increase in the number of people suffering digestive issues and diseases. Digestive imbalances can manifest themselves in many forms, from the severe cases of Crohn's, colitis and leaky gut, to undiagnosed IBS, chronic fatigue and candida overgrowth. Although not all of these conditions can be cured by diet alone, eating well-balanced, nutritionally-dense foods helps to heal and support digestion in its daily functioning. As a long-term sufferer of post-infectious IBS, I have first hand experience of the improvements the body feels when it is given the correct foods it needs for its optimal functioning.

the mouth

The mouth is the first step in the digestive process. Chewing food thoroughly breaks down the larger pieces of food into smaller particles, making it easier for our stomach to breakdown. It is also where food is first exposed to amylase, an enzyme created by the salivary glands, which assists in breaking down food, contributing to the overall chemical process of digestion.

small mouthfuls

There is a 20 minute window whilst eating before our brain signals to our stomachs that we are full. Eating slowly, with smaller mouthfuls, gives the body time to work out whether it is full, and can prevent accidental overeating.

chewing food

I don't advocate any specific number of times you should chew food, as ultimately you should take an approach that works best for you. When chewing your food, try not to think of the number of times you have chewed it, but instead the enjoyment of eating it. Chewing your food completely until it is small enough to be swallowed with ease will help you get a sense of your own eating patterns and help you develop a relationship with the food you consume. The saliva produced when chewing also relaxes the lower stomach (pylorus) muscles, aiding the food's progress through your stomach and into your small intestine.

the stomach

The next stage of the digestive process takes place in the stomach, where a hormone called gastrin (which relates to acid secretion) is produced in response to the presence of food. The acid in the stomach is responsible for killing off bacteria and other micro-organisms that enter the body with food. It also breaks down proteins, activates digestive enzymes, and facilitates later absorption in the intestine. Part of successfully "cooking" the food in the stomach requires having a balanced level of acidity.

stomach acidity test

First thing in the morning, before eating or drinking anything, mix ¼ teaspoon bicarbonate of soda in 200ml cold water. Drink the solution and time how long it takes for you to start burping. If your stomach is producing adequate amounts of hydrochloric acid, you will burp within 2–3 minutes. Early or repeated belching is due to an excessive amount of stomach acid.

high acidity

Often, excessively high or low stomach acidity display very similar symptoms, such as heartburn, gastric ulcers and acid reflux, so it is important to correctly identify which the problem is, in order to prevent inappropriate treatment. Try to identify foods that contribute to excess stomach acid and aid the healing by eating natural anti-inflammatory foods such as ginger, turmeric and mineral-rich greens and vegetables. Eliminate salty, spicy, highly processed (pre-made) food, sugar, alcohol and caffeinated foods. Remember, if your body has gone off balance, it takes time for it to return to its equilibrium, so be patient and allow it to take the time it needs.

low acidity
When the pH is high (and the acid level low), food takes longer to digest, which can result in fermentation and issues with bacterial overgrowth. There are many natural ways to increase the natural production of stomach acid: try mixing a tablespoon of raw apple cider vinegar with a couple of tablespoons of warm water and drinking it first thing in the morning, 15 minutes before eating. Another method is drinking a large glass of water before meals. Contrary to popular belief, drinking water before meals actually triggers the production of stomach acid. The water prepares the body for food, prompting the intestine to produce mucus to protect the intestine from the stomach acid, thus allowing the stomach to make more acid and "cook" the food properly.

sensitive stomach
When the stomach feels weak, it is advisable to eat foods that are easily digestible. Avoiding excessive consumption of raw fruits and vegetables during times of more sensitive digestion is advisable, as the plant cell walls are made of cellulose fibres that the human digestive system struggles to break down. When uncooked, these cell walls are harder for the body to

break down and requires more energy. Warm and nourishing soups and rice-based dishes like the yoga bowl (see page 26) and drinks like turmeric latte (see page 105) are soothing options.

cleansing foods
sea salt Although salt should be used in careful moderation, a little can have beneficial effects. High mineral sea salt stimulates acid production in the stomach.
lemon Drinking hot water with fresh lemon throughout the day is cleansing for the stomach, as it acts as a natural detoxificant and decongestant. It is beneficial to drink first thing in the morning, before eating, to prepare the stomach for food.
ginger Ginger is a natural digestive and can be used to treat various types of stomach ailments. Try making an infusion with lemon and hot water, juicing it, or blending into smoothies.

healing foods
miso soup Made from fermented soy beans, it acts as a natural probiotic due to the micro-organisms used in the fermentation process. It also contains a high number of easily absorbable zinc (good for immunity) and manganese (assists the thyroid and regulates metabolic rate).
oats A neutral, plain-tasting food, oats are best eaten in the form of porridge, to soothe the stomach. They are also high in beneficial vitamins and minerals and a good source of fibre.
brown rice Washed thoroughly and cooked properly, rice makes a good stomach soother because it is neutral and so doesn't irritate the stomach. It is also a good

source of fibre.

the intestine
Made up of the large and the small intestine, this organ is one of the largest and most complex in our bodies. The intestinal tract relies on the presence of beneficial bacteria to support its specialised immune-supporting cells and a complex network of neurological and hormonal components. It acts as the headquarters for immunity and neurological health, housing the tools for breaking down food and also numerous nerve endings and sensors that relate directly to our immune, hormonal and nervous systems. The gut is also home to the largest concentration of mood-altering neurotransmitters, with around 80% of our serotonin receptors.

a note on IBS
Having tried many different diets, the one I have found most useful in easing symptoms of IBS is the low FODMAP diet. It advocates the restriction of all highly fermentable short-chain carbohydrates that are often poorly digested in the small intestine, causing rapid fermentation in the gut, exacerbating the symptoms of IBS. The research is relatively new and being developed all the time. If IBS is something you suffer with, it is certainly a diet to look into (under the guidance of a registered dietitian).

cleansing foods, spices + herbs
grapefruit Grapefruit is rich in dietary insoluble fibre pectin, which, by acting as a bulk laxative, helps to protect the colon mucus membrane by

decreasing exposure time to toxic substancesin the colon. It also facilitates dietary iron absorption from the intestine. Eat whole or use the juice for smoothies and freshly squeezed juices.

turmeric The yellow or orange pigment of turmeric, curcumin has long been used as a treatment for inflammatory bowel disease (IBD), such as Crohn's and ulcerative colitis. It is a beneficial ingredient for a number of dishes from curries, to dressings, and is also delicious as a tea.

oily fish They reduce inflammation and help in healing the digestive tract lining. They can also improve nutrient absorption, help balance hormones, improve neurological function and boost immunity.

healing spices + herbs

peppermint The ultimate herb to stimulate the flow of digestive juices and ease cramps. Add to salads, salsas and Asian dishes, or infuse the leaves in hot water for a digestive soothing tea.

fennel An effective digestive and anti spasmodic, fennel aids bloating, heartburn and gas. It can be eaten both raw in salads and cooked.

cultured fermented foods

Fermented food is known to support the balance of beneficial bacteria in the gut. These include foods like kimchi and sauerkraut, both made of fermented cabbage (page 32) and also miso soup, from fermented soy beans.

energy detox

what is the energy detox?

The entire focus of this cleanse is geared towards improving the body's energy generation system. Rarely have I ever found a diet where the reports proclaim anything other than tiredness, loss of energy and lack of motivation. Usually this is due to an insufficient amount of calories. When we are detoxing and cleansing the system, the body needs fuel to work properly.

We often need look no further than the quality of food in our daily meals to see the association between food and fatigue. Just think about the heavy distended feeling you have after eating a large meal. Food should fill us with vitality and energy, not make us want to pass out. The energy cleanse focuses on the foods that do just that, by removing the things we rely on for social energy (namely alcohol, sugar and caffeine), emphasising the key foods that stimulate the organs responsible for rebooting our energy stores, and encouraging toxin elimination.

why do the detox?

When we are feeling low and energy-depleted, it is too easy to rely on borrowed energy, in the form of either caffeine, sugar, nicotine or alcohol. In the short run they keep our bodies ticking over, but in the long run they impair the adrenals, kidney and liver, and we find ourselves in a spiral of continual fatigue. Stimulant foods and drinks are also acid-forming and break down the body's resistance and immunity.

When enjoyed in moderation and as part of a balanced diet, these foods are not necessarily a negative thing. In fact, they can be quite positive; coffee is known to improve brain cognitive function and increase the amount of dopamine released by the brain. Red wine is also known to be high in resveratrol, a beneficial "heart healthy" antioxidant found in very few foods. It is only once the body becomes reliant upon them that they become a problem. Stimulation requires re-stimulation to alleviate the downswing of the initial indulgence.

Having experienced the effects of caffeine and sugar dependence first hand, I fully understand how all-consuming they can be and how giving them up, or even cutting them right back, can seem impossible. In truth, sometimes it gets a little bit harder before it gets easier. This is why giving them up, full stop, for these five days is key. It's just a chance to give the body a well-deserved break and to help restore the body with healing foods and drinks that rebalance the organs most responsible for keeping you energised and awake.

a note about salt

An excess of sodium encourages our cells to store water, giving the body a heavy, sluggish feeling. During this time of detox, cut your salt intake right back; you will certainly notice the difference. In place of added salt, you can use herbs and spices to enhance the flavours in dishes.

liver

One of the largest organs in the body, the liver mainly acts as a filter for the blood coming from the digestive tract, passing it to the rest of the body. It also performs many essential functions related to digestion, metabolism, immunity and the storage of nutrients within the body. This includes: storing glycogen (fuel for the body); processing fats and proteins from digested food, and processing medicines and chemicals; removing poisons and toxins taken in by the body.

what it is affected by
Enzymes in the liver are responsible for metabolising alcohol, sugar and drugs. A poor diet, unhealthy weight, lack of exercise and high cholesterol are all factors that directly affect its capacity to function.

cut out the chemicals
Any harmful chemicals, pesticides and other food sprays that your intestine cannot digest are passed through to the liver to process. Not only are they harmful for the function of the liver in the short term, but over longer periods of time they can build up in the body, causing disease and longer-term health issues. Although our exposure to chemicals cannot be removed completely, here are a few ways of reducing your intake:
• Source organic or higher welfare meat, dairy and eggs wherever possible. Buy the best you can afford.
• Wash all fruit and vegetables thoroughly before using, especially if they are non-organic.
• Buy a water filter; even just a water bottle with a filter is useful to help purify your water when you are on the go.
• Switch your cleaning sprays and soaps to natural products.

• Limit excessive consumption of fructose foods as the body cannot assimilate fructose and an excess of it leads to fat build-up in the liver.

cleansing foods, spices + herbs
broccoli It contains a phytochemical called sulforaphane, which is a natural inducer of the liver's detoxifying system.
green tea A plant full of antioxidants known as catechins, known to assist liver function.
turmeric A powerful anti-inflammatory used to treat a wide variety of conditions.

healing foods, spices + herbs
avocado It stimulates the production of glutathione, an essential nutrient for liver health.
cinnamon This helps support the liver by reducing the triglyceride response after eating.

kidneys

The role of the kidneys is to balance the pH levels and salt in the blood, to keep blood composition levels constant. It is their job to remove excess water and waste liquids, which get secreted from your kidneys as urine. If your kidneys are not functioning properly, accumulated waste can build up in both the kidneys and the blood.

what they are affected by High blood pressure can damage blood vessels in the kidneys, reducing their ability to work properly. If these blood vessels get damaged, they become less able to remove waste and fluids from the body, which in turn can increase blood pressure levels further. Unlike the stomach and

intestines, food never sees the kidneys, so they are only affected on a secondary level.

cleansing foods, spices + herbs
go veggie for a day Instead of eating meat daily, try going vegetarian for two days a week. A vegetable/fruit-based diet allows the body system to alkalinise via the kidneys.
parsley An important diuretic, parsley helps clear uric acid from the urinary tract and helps dissolve and expel gallstones and gravel.
dandelion leaves + roots These have been used for centuries to treat liver, gall bladder, kidney and joint problems. They are also a natural source of potassium, and will replenish any that may be lost due to the diuretic action of the other kidney-cleaning herbs, such as parsley and marshmallow root.
marshmallow root It has a directly soothing effect on inflamed and irritated tissues of the alimentary canal, and urinary and respiratory organs. It also has factors which eliminate toxins, helping the body to cleanse.

healing foods, spices + herbs
chamomile Anti-inflammatory and eases pain, infection and allergy, most commonly cystitis.
cranberry Commonly used to help prevent and treat urinary tract infections, it also helps to kill germs and speed skin healing.
nettles These contain natural anti-inflammatory properties and also stimulates urinary release and the expulsion of water from the body, helping to flush bacteria out of the urinary tract.

adrenals

The adrenal glands manage adrenaline production and regulate blood sugar levels. They are also affected when a person is under stress, and if a person is in a constant state of physical or emotional stress, the adrenals become fatigued and stop functioning optimally. This is known as adrenal fatigue or exhaustion.

what they are affected by

Caffeine and sugar both have a big effect on the adrenal glands, stimulating them and giving the body a short-term booster of mental and physical energy, which makes us feel more able and motivated. This injection of energy is an over-exertion that the body has to make up for afterwards. When our adrenal glands are constantly required to sustain high adrenaline levels, they eventually become impaired in their ability to respond appropriately. It is adrenaline that is responsible for the little burst of energy that wakes us up in the morning, and for keeping us awake, alert and focused throughout the rest of the day. Needless to say, these glands are crucial to our health and symptoms of adrenal fatigue include tiredness that is not relieved by sleep, salt cravings, difficulty focusing, poor memory and inability to cope with stress. The adrenals are also affected by emotional stress.

vitamins + herbs to rebalance the adrenals

vitamin C A critical vitamin for stress reduction and adrenal health, vitamin C is used by the adrenal glands in the production of all of the adrenal hormones, most notably cortisol. In adrenal fatigue, your adrenal glands release more cortisol when faced with a vitamin C deficiency. This increases immediate anxiety and prolongs a state of high cortisol, which is bad for blood sugar and blood pressure, and contributes to the storing of fat in the body.

magnesium Magnesium plays a role in the function of more than 300 enzymes in the human body. When you are magnesium-deficient, the point at which your adrenals kick in to produce their fight-or-flight hormone is lower. Eating food high in magnesium can help improve this.

ashwagandha + ginseng Both of these are good adaptogens, which help the adrenals adjust to stress. They are also both potent antioxidants, help improve immune function and work to decrease anxiety.

liquorice It supports the production of cortisol and has long been used to support adrenal health. It supports the immune system and helps ease fatigue, pain and weakness associated with adrenal depletion.

detox note

If you do feel you are suffering from any of the symptoms outlined in this text, do seek out the help of a registered doctor, dietitian or nutritionist for a full diagnosis.

the naked storecupboard

Although I tend to let fresh produce dictate the base of most of my meals, I always keep my storecupboards stocked with natural 'naked' essentials – ingredients I can reach for to produce the recipes I love to eat and cook on a daily basis. Having a well-stocked storecupboard means always being prepared, and gives any cook flexibility and a reliable ingredient source to work from.

Throughout the years, my storecupboard has seen many ingredients come and go. Freekeh, bulgar, barberries, you name it. I am always interested in trying every new and unpronounceable grain, flour, noodle or spice that crosses my path.

Despite my excitement for new finds, if you were to open my storecupboards on any given day, you would always find a selection of key, foundation items – the naked backbone of my cooking. Most of the ingredients I use are readily available in most larger supermarkets, but unfortunately many local smaller spots don't tend to stock kamut flour or farro grains. I can't for the life of me think why not… it would serve the world a whole lot better if they swapped the bright magpie-luring confectionery for hearty wholegrains. So it just takes a little preparation, a bit of an online shop, or a trip to a slightly larger supermarket every now and then.

In the process of writing this book, I did a lot of research with family and friends, asking them where they felt they would like to improve their diet and what their main obstacles were in acheiving it. One of the most recurring answers that came up was habit and routine. Having a well-stocked storecupboard makes it that much easier to choose healthier options when it comes to daily dishes. Even the cook with the best of intentions can be lured by the quick-cook, refined variety when its wholegrain counterpart is not available.

In an attempt to move away from the processed, refined and abundant quantity of bleached white foods that line so many storecupboards, here is a list of naked alternatives. These are the staple, unprocessed, unrefined 'naked' ingredients that are the foundations of **the naked diet**.

a brief overview on gluten-free, dairy-free + sugar-free

To clarify, this book is not strictly oriented towards any specific health-related diet. It is naturally low in carbohydrates, free from processed food and contains no refined sugar, but it is not gluten-free, dairy-free or vegan (although many of the recipes can be adapted to accommodate these).

flours

The more familiar varieties of flour are made from grains and cereals (such as wheat, spelt and rye) but flours are also made from ground pulses, nuts, fruits and seeds. One thing to consider when choosing a flour is what you are intending to use it for, as the way one flour functions is different to another, and it's not as simple as substituting one kind for another.

spelt An ancient ground wheat flour, with a lower GI and a higher profile of nutrients, spelt contains gluten, but in lower quantities than traditional wheat. It is easier to digest than most grains and is recommended as a wheat alternative to sufferers of poor digestion and irritable gut. It can be bought either white or wholegrain, has a nutty taste and can be used for making breads and for baking.

rye Naturally lower in gluten than wheat, rye has a rich deep flavour. It is best to buy it milled from whole grains of rye which are stone ground. Although it contains gluten, it tends to give heavy results, so when baking use it mixed with other flours, which lightens the flavour and gives a better rise.

kamut Also known as khorasan flour, kamut is another ancient wheat flour, originally grown for the pharaohs in Egypt. It is naturally high in protein and minerals such as selenium. It has a higher level of gluten than spelt and is good for homemade pasta and bread.

gluten-free Gluten-free flour can be made from any variety of non-gluten containing food. Mostly these are not grains, but legumes, seeds or nuts. Most of the advertised 'gluten-free flour' you see on the shelves of supermarkets is the processed white variety, which has a high GI, is low in nutrition and contains little fibre. I tend to buy brown rice or buckwheat flour.

semolina/polenta This is a grainy meal made from coarsely ground corn. It is best to buy stoneground, as the hull and germ are still attached, giving it more flavour and a higher nutritional value.

cornflour This is the only white flour I allow in my storecupboard, and then only to be used in small amounts. It is the powdered starch of the maize grain, and although it lacks the beneficial husk and germ of the corn, its fineness makes it a useful, gluten-free thickening agent.

almond Usually made from ground, blanched almonds, this is a favourite for grain-free and low-carb baking. It is high in omega-3 fats. I like to buy whole, unblanched almonds and grind my own in a high-speed blender, to store in a sealed jar.

coconut A good gluten-free, low-carb, nut-free flour alternative, coconut flour, contains more dietary fibre than other wheat alternatives, and is naturally high in beneficial fats.

brown rice + buckwheat Both of these are gluten-free and often used in baking. They can be used alone, but work best when combined with other flours. Although from different sources, they yield similar results in cooking and are interchangeable.

sugars

Natural sugars have a lower GI than processed refined sugar, and contain more beneficial nutrients. As with flour, I generally steer clear of anything white, and keep a range of different types in the storecupboard for varying flavours. There are a lot of sugars and sweeteners to be wary of. High fructose sugars, like agave or 'fruit-based' sweeteners, are often marketed as a healthy sugar alternative, when actually they are highly processed, poorly digested and cause a strain on the liver.

maple syrup Made from the sap of maple trees, this naturally occurring sugar has a lower GI than honey.

honey Another natural source of sugar, honey is known for its healing properties, especially manuka honey from New Zealand and Australia. Always buy raw honey, as it hasn't been heated or processed in any way and will have all the enzymes intact. I recommend avoiding cooking with honey, or heating it to over 40°C, because it will change its molecular structure.

coconut palm sugar Also called jaggery, this is available in granulated form, has a much lower GI than regular cane sugar and makes for a great alternative for healthy baking. It's rich and treacly in flavour, like soft brown sugar.

blackstrap molasses Molasses is the dark, syrupy by-product from the process of sugar extraction from sugarcane. It is important to buy organic and unsulphured, which contains all the minerals and nutrients absorbed by the sugar cane.

liquid stevia Another natural sweetener, with no calories and no impact on GI, stevia is therefore suitable for diabetics and is available in a range of different flavours. It is best in liquid form, I like vanilla, and often substitute half of another variety of sugar for stevia. 1 drop is as sweet as 1 teaspoon coconut palm sugar.

grains + pulses

Not only are grains and pulses cheap and delicious, they also contain a lot of beneficial nutrients that are overlooked when we condemn their ground, milled over-used counterparts. I like to have at least one day a week without eating meat, and find grain-based dishes the most satisfying and filling. As they are in their whole form, they are much lower in GI, and higher in fibre. Eaten in combination with fresh, seasonal vegetables, roasted nuts and fresh herbs, these grains and pulses form the foundation of some of my favourite dishes.

pearl barley Not to be confused with wholegrain barley, this is the barley grain with the bran and hull removed. It takes on a creamy texture when cooked and can be used in place of rice in risottos.

farro + spelt Farro is a whole grain often used in Italian cooking that looks similar to pearl barley but has a nuttier flavour. It retains its shape when cooked, so works best in salads. Spelt is also known as dinkel wheat, wheat berries or hulled wheat. Both are useful ingredients and are pretty interchangeable between dishes.

red rice Usually from the Camargue region of France, this short-grained rice has a slightly nutty taste and chewy texture.

brown basmati A variety of long-grain rice from the Indian subcontinent, brown basmati still contains its husk. It is high in fibre and beneficial vitamins and can be used in place of white rice.

quinoa This South American seed is often denoted for its high protein and low carbohydrate levels. It is a good gluten-free alternative to grain and has a range of different colours. I favour the dramatic black and red varieties in appearance, although the cooking time and taste of each is very similar.

chickpeas One of the most versatile legumes, chickpeas are a useful staple to have on hand for quick salads, stews, soups or dips. They are high in protein and low in fat, making them a good meat substitute. Buying dried is best, but cooking requires soaking so if time is an issue, opt for the tinned variety, preferring organic.

cannellini + butter beans High in protein and low in fat, both varieties of white bean are very mild in flavour and thus a versatile staple. Dried are best but require soaking.

red lentils There are many lentil varieties, the red being best for making dhals, curries and stews, as they are lower in fibre then the puy variety. 30% of their calories are from protein, making them the third highest protein source of any legume or nut. They also have a high iron content.

puy lentils Another variety of lentil, puy holds its shape when cooked, making it good for salads. It is best to soak them before use; not only does this reduce the cooking time, it also reduces a natural, non-digestible phytic acid which often can lead to digestive discomfort.

fruits, nuts + seeds

dates Best bought dried, dates are a sweet, edible fruit. They are high in fibre and a number of vitamins and minerals, and are useful for bringing sweetness to savoury dishes, as well as to smoothies and puddings.

sultanas + raisins Both are a type of dried grape, these can be used in anything from baking to smoothies. Soaking them in liquid before using plumps them up.

dried cherries + currants These are tarter and tend to be a little smaller than sultanas and raisins. They are very versatile, I use them in savoury dishes, such as rice salads.

goji berries High in antioxidants and minerals, these dried berries have been used in Chinese medicine for years. They are less sweet than raisins, but without the tartness of sour cherries. I add them to granola, smoothies and salads, for colour and texture.

almonds One of the most popular and versatile of nuts, almonds make a great storecupboard staple. Best bought whole, unpeeled and raw, you can roast them, or blitz them into milk or flour; they are also good to have on hand for a healthy snack.

cashews One of the milder flavoured nuts, cashews have a high oil content, which means they blend very well into a thick, creamy texture. They are ideal for making nut butter. As they are high in mould, anyone suffering from issues with candida in the gut is advised to avoid eating cashews.

hazelnuts One of my two favourite nuts, hazelnuts are undoubtedly at their best when toasted. I tend to buy them in autumn (often in their shell) and crack them myself. They find their way into anything from wintry salads, to granola, nut milks and smoothies.

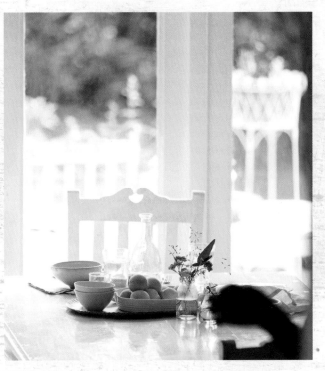

desiccated + flaked coconut
Made from the flesh of the coconut, but processed for different effects, these are gluten-free and have a low GI. Desiccated results in small flecks, with flaked tending to be slightly larger. Both are great additions to baking, or can be simply sprinkled over yoghurt or porridge at breakfast time.

spices + herbs

Spices are a wonderful way to pack complex flavours into simple dishes. They often have a lot of health benefits in their own right and have been used for years in traditional medicines to treat ailments and support good health, especially in the digestive tract. It is best to buy spices whole and grind them yourself, in small batches, as they lose their potency after a few months. Herbs are very much a subjective choice, depending on the foods and cuisines you tend to gravitate towards in your cooking.

cinnamon With its naturally sweet taste, cinnamon is one of the most popular spices in baking. It can be bought in stick form or ground and stays fresh for longer when bought whole, but ground is certainly more convenient. Cinnamon is known to aid digestion and helps to fight bacterial infections.

cardamom This aromatic spice comes in different varieties, most recognisable as a small seed encased in a green pod. They are best bought in whole pods and ground down, to retain freshness. Cardamom can ease indigestion and excess stomach acid.

cayenne pepper Found in ground form, from a South

pistachios Often used in Middle Eastern cooking, pistachios add a delicious flavour and a lovely pop of colour to so many sweet and savoury dishes. They are also a member of the cashew family and, as such, can also be mould-forming and not advisable for people with candida.

pecans My other favourite nut, pecans are sweet, rich, complex in flavour and can be easily bought whole, halved or chopped. Undoubtedly at their best when toasted, they work wonders with sweet-tasting ingredients, especially chocolate, maple syrup and sweet potatoes.

mixed seeds The variety of seeds I have varies. Sometimes it is a mixed jar of linseed, sunflower and pumpkin. Generally they are interchangeable, but a mixed selection is always best.

pine nuts Slightly more expensive than other nuts, with a high oil content and a unique flavour, pine nuts make a classic addition to salads, but also work superbly well in sweet dishes too. I like to pair them with dried cranberries in my nut butter bars.

sesame seeds Small and intense in flavour, these make a great addition to Asian dishes. I often have a pot of them toasted by my cooker to add a sprinkle to finish off dishes, and they work well as a mild-flavoured nut milk.

chia seeds Small and black, these look like poppy seeds and are one of the highest vegetarian sources of omega-3 fatty acids. When soaked, they break down and become gelatinous, making them ideal for baking and smoothies. However, they are not ideal for toasting or sprinkling on salads.

American variety of hot red pepper, cayenne is used to add heat and spice to dishes. It also helps the body to flush out toxins, and stimulates weight loss by boosting metabolism.

chilli flakes These are a dried and crushed version of the red chilli with seeds, most commonly made from ancho bell or cayenne pepper. They add heat and flavour, but also colour to dishes. Chilli is also known to improve blood circulation and boost energy levels.

coriander seeds These dried berries of the coriander herb have a deeper, different taste to the fresh stalks and leaves. For best results, buy them whole and grind them yourself. Unlike any other spice, they are a source of vitamin C.

cumin seeds The seeds of a small plant related to the parsley family, these have a distinctive earthy flavour, commonly used in Middle Eastern and Indian cooking. For best results, buy them whole and grind them yourself.

nutmeg Whole nutmegs come as small egg-shaped seeds, and have a rich, slightly sweet taste. For best results, buy them whole and grate them. Nutmeg contains two compounds called myristicin and elemicin, both known to stimulate mental activity.

saffron The most expensive spice, obtained from the stamen of a crocus, saffron is mild in flavour, so other spices should be used lightly so as not to mask it. It also gives food a wonderful yellow colour.

smoked paprika Made from capsicum annuum pepper, smoked paprika can be smooth, sweet or spicy depending on the variety. I buy both a Spanish spicy variety and the sweet, smoky sort as well. It adds a wonderful richness and depth to dishes and dressings.

kaffir lime leaves A popular ingredient in south east Asian cooking, these are best bought and used fresh, but having a dried pot is handy for times when they are hard to come by. They add a distinctive, floral freshness and vibrancy to soups, curries and pastes.

bay leaves Whenever I find a bay tree, I pick a large handful of leaves and leave them in a warm place to dry out. They are useful for adding depth of flavour and richness to meat, soups and stews, as well as to sweet dishes. Try infusing a couple of leaves in your milk especially when making hot chocolate.

dried rosemary Useful for flavouring, rosemary is a popular herb in many dishes. Try drying branches of rosemary yourself, by tying one end with string and leaving in a warm place to dry out. Break off the leaves and store in sealed containers for handy use.

dried thyme Another popular herb for flavouring dishes, thyme can be dried in the same way as rosemary.

oils + condiments

Oils can be extracted from a number of different sources. The best ones to use are those with minimal processing, which more often than not means cold-pressed, extra virgin and organic oils. These oils have been produced in a way to retain the highest amount of nutritional components possible, and are beneficial for good health.

There are three categories of fat: saturated, monounsaturated and polyunsaturated. Saturated fats are made up of solely saturated triglycerides (fat), and are most commonly found in dairy products. They tend to harden to a solid at room temperature. Coconut oil and ghee are both grouped as a 'saturated fat', and although saturates are often condemned as bad, this is not strictly the case, as both of these have many health benefits and remain stable at higher cooking temperatures. Monounsaturated fats are long-chain fats that remain liquid at room temperature. They have a thicker viscosity than polyunsaturates, which makes them more suited to use in cooking. Polyunsaturates, on the other hand, have a very thin viscosity at all temperatures. They also have a delicate molecular structure, so are not ideal to cook with and are better used to finish dishes, or in dressings.

virgin coconut oil Coconut oil is extracted from the kernel or meat of matured coconuts. It is great for cooking with as unlike other oils, it remains stable at high temperatures. However, because it is a saturated fat it sets hard at room temperature and has a mild, sweet coconut flavour that isn't ideal for dressings. It has a whole host of health benefits, including boosting metabolism and is a source of the powerful antiviral and antibacterial lauric acid.

ghee This is clarified butter, made by extracting the oil and discarding the milk solids from butter. It is about two-thirds a saturated fat, which means it remains stable at higher temperatures. This makes it ideal for pan-frying and sautéing in place of butter, giving dishes that wonderful, rich buttery flavour without the risk of burning the milk solids in butter.

extra virgin olive oil My favourite of all oils, this is the highest quality and most expensive olive oil. It is suitable for cooking, but only at low temperatures. I love the distinctive grassy notes and often use it as a condiment or in dressings. It is best to buy fresh pressed and organic.

infused oils Infusing oils is quick and easy to do and I always have a bottle of garlic oil on the go. I tend to do this with a lesser quality, but still organic, olive oil, as it has a milder flavour and takes on the taste of the infusing ingredient better. It is suitable for cooking, but at low temperatures only.

toasted sesame oil This rich, strong-flavoured oil is extracted from toasted sesame seeds. It is not a stable oil to cook with and is best used as a condiment or dressing. As it is very distinctive in flavour, it is best used sparingly.

balsamic vinegar The king of all vinegars, I am never without a bottle of good-quality balsamic. Like olive oil, you get what you pay for, and it is worth investing in a higher quality variety. It adds richness and sweetness as well as a vinegary kick to dishes.

raw apple cider vinegar It is best to buy raw and unfiltered cider vinegar as it has the beneficial living enzymes in the vinegar. This variety is alkaline-forming in the body and known for its nutrients and health benefits.

Dijon mustard The traditional French, creamy, pale yellow mustard, Dijon is lighter than the English variety.

tamari Tamari is a Japanese form of soy sauce, traditionally made as a by-product of miso paste. It tastes a lot like soy sauce, but is often gluten-free.

fish sauce An amber-coloured liquid extracted from the fermentation of anchovies with sea salt, it is used in Asian cooking.

rosewater Made from a distillate of rose petals, rosewater is a by-product from rose oil used in the manufacture of perfume. Particularly popular in Middle Eastern food, it adds a floral taste and can be used in both savoury and sweet dishes.

orange blossom water Distilled from orange blossom, this has a very distinctive and refreshing citrus-floral flavour. It is quite strong and should be used sparingly.

tahini A rich paste made from ground, hulled sesame seeds, tahini is essentially sesame seed butter. I use it in anything, including dips, dressings and even smoothies.

nut butter This form of spreadable nuts can be bought or made, and used in a vast number of dishes. All types offer different benefits in terms of taste and health. The most versatile are certainly almond, cashew and peanut butter, and these tend to be the ones I buy.

chywanaprash This jam-like, cooked mixture of honey, ghee, tryphala and many other herbs and spices is used in Ayurvedic medicine as a supplement. It can also be added to hot drinks, such as honey and lemon.

cereals

There are vast numbers of different grains, flakes and cereals on the market. For the sake of storage space and necessity I try to keep my storecupboard condensed into a few key essentials. Most health food stores will stock them and, if not, they can be found online.

oats A staple cereal grain that I use practically daily in savoury and sweet dishes, oats are a slow release carbohydrate, filled with fibre. They can be bought gluten-free too.

buckwheat groats These are raw, unprocessed buckwheat kernels that can be roasted or sprouted. They are naturally gluten-free and make a great addition to granola and muesli.

spelt flakes I often use these as a substitute for oats in dishes when I am looking for a richer flavour. As the spelt grain is related to wheat, it does contain a small amount of gluten, but is easily digestible.

quinoa flakes Made from unprocessed, flattened quinoa seeds, these are high in protein and beneficial omega-3 fatty acids, and are also lower in carbohydrates than most grains. They can be used in anything from breakfast to baking, and are naturally gluten-free.

superfoods

A lot of hype surrounds superfoods and their benefits. Although there is no guarantee that eating superfoods will drastically change your health, they are all mineral- and vitamin-rich and, as such, can make a beneficial addition to the diet.

maca This root is also called Peruvian ginseng and has an earthy, deep caramel flavour.

Most commonly available in powder form, it is known to improve energy and boost vitality and libido in both men and women.

raw cacao Raw cacao is made by cold pressing unroasted cocoa beans, a process that preserves the living enzymes in the cocoa. Raw cacao is also high in resveratrol, an antioxidant that helps protect the nervous system. It can be bought as nibs or ground.

spirulina This type of blue-green algae, most commonly bought in powder form, is largely made up of protein and essential amino acids. It can be added to juices and smoothies, but sparingly, as it is not the most pleasant-tasting of superfoods.

chlorella Another variety of blue-green algae available in powder form, chlorella contains the highest levels of chlorophyll found in any edible plant. Its taste is even less appetising than spirulina, so may be best taken in tablet form, rather then used as a powdered ingredient.

wheatgrass The pressed leaf of the wheat plant, wheatgrass is often supplied freshly made, but can also be bought in powder form. It is a much sweeter-tasting green superfood and gives dishes and smoothies a vibrant green colour.

lucuma A naturally sweet sub-tropical fruit native to the Andean valleys of Peru, lucuma makes a delicious addition to shakes, smoothies and puddings. It is also nice simply stirred through yoghurt and served with fresh berries.

baobab Originating from the tree of the same name in Africa, baobab is 50% fibre and is extremely high in vitamin C and beneficial B vitamins. It has a distinct, citrussy taste and is best used stirred into porridge and sprinkled on cereal.

mesquite Another South American superfood, extracted from the pods of the mesquite tree, mesquite is high in fibre and calcium. It has a rich, spiced flavour, a little like a combination of coffee, cacao and cinnamon, and is best for sweet dishes and smoothies.

bee pollen This is the pollen packed by worker honeybees into small granules with the added nectar, and is very high in amino acids. It has a pleasing sweet taste, and works as a good natural sweetener for smoothies and raw puddings.

reishi mushrooms They are a herbal mushroom used in Chinese medicine and one of the oldest to be used medicinally. They are high in antioxidants, good for boosting the immune system and are thought to fight the growth of cancerous cells. They are bitter in taste, so best bought dried as a powder or as tablets.

ashwagandha Made from Indian winter cherry, this is one of the most beneficial herbs in Ayurvedic medicine, known for its restorative benefits and immune system support. It has an earthy, bonfire, bitter taste.

shatavari Derived from a variety of asparagus, this other beneficial herb in Ayurvedic medicine is commonly used to support the female reproductive system. It can help with mood swings and PMS, as well as menopausal hot flashes. It can be bought as a powder and has a sweet and bitter taste.

index

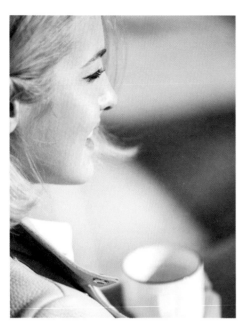

Acknowledgments

To my parents who have supported me, Fred who loved me and Humphrey who cured me. Also all the wonderful support from the brilliant minds of all my wonderful friends, editors, agents, students and teachers. Thank you for keeping me inspired.

This is a book for all the budding cooks, food lovers and aspiring healthy eaters. It is a way to live, love and eat today and everyday. With real, unprocessed and 'naked' foods.

I hope it makes you as happy to read and cook as it made me to write and taste.

With love
Tess x

Publishing director: Sarah Lavelle
Creative director: Helen Lewis
Editor: Romilly Morgan
Copy editor: Sally Somers
Design: Katherine Keeble
Photography: Columbus Leth
Food stylist: Rukmini Iyer
Props stylist: Rachel Jukes
Production: Vincent Smith, Stephen Lang

First published in 2015 by Quadrille Publishing Limited

Text © 2015 Tess Ward
Photography © 2015 Columbus Leth
Design and layout © 2015 Quadrille Publishing Limited

Quadrille is an imprint of Hardie Grant www.hardiegrant.com.au

Quadrille Publishing Ltd
Pentagon House
52–54 Southwark Street
London SE1 1UN
www.quadrille.co.uk

Cataloguing in Publication Data: a catalogue record for this book is available from the British Library.

ISBN: 978 1 84949 604 9

Printed in China